VISUAL
ERGONOMICS
HANDBOOK

VISUAL ERGONOMICS

HANDBOOK

EDITED BY

JEFFREY ANSHEL

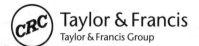

Taylor & Francis
Taylor & Francis Group

Boca Raton   London   New York   Singapore

A CRC title, part of the Taylor & Francis imprint, a member of the
Taylor & Francis Group, the academic division of T&F Informa plc.

Published in 2005 by
CRC Press
Taylor & Francis Group
6000 Broken Sound Parkway NW, Suite 300
Boca Raton, FL 33487-2742

International Standard Book Number-10: 1-56670-682-3 (Hardcover)
International Standard Book Number-13: 978-1-56670-682-7 (Hardcover)
Library of Congress Card Number 2005041779

Library of Congress Cataloging-in-Publication Data

Visual ergonomics handbook / edited by Jeffrey Anshel.
    p. cm.
ISBN 1-56670-682-3 (alk. paper)
1. Vision--Handbooks, manuals, etc. 2. Vision disorders--Handbooks, manuals, etc. 3. Video display terminals--Health aspects--Handbooks, manuals, etc. 4. Human-computer interaction-- Handbooks, manuals, etc.

RC965.V53V57 2005
617.7--dc22   2005041779

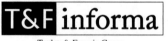

Taylor & Francis Group
is the Academic Division of T&F Informa plc.

Visit the Taylor & Francis Web site at
http://www.taylorandfrancis.com

and the CRC Press Web site at
http://www.crcpress.com

Contents

Preface

If you are reading this book clearly and comfortably, then congratulations — your eyes are probably working well. Yet it's also most likely that you spend several hours per day staring at a computer screen (maybe even while reading this book). Viewing an electronic display screen varies significantly from reading text on paper and our eyes most often suffer for it. We need to address this problem and find out what can be done to make our computer viewing time more comfortable, as well as more productive.

Both optometrists and ergonomists realize that the eyes are a critical part of proper ergonomics. It has been said that the eyes lead the body, so one cannot rightfully be considered without the other. However, ergonomists often have just a rudimentary understanding of the human visual system. This text combines the efforts of leading experts in the fields of optometry, ergonomics, eye safety, and occupational medicine. It integrates their knowledge into a comprehensive, easy-to-read volume that is sure to appeal to all interested parties.

The first chapters deal with the eyes and visual system. Chapter 1 starts off with a historical perspective on how our vision and visual system are designed to work and how they have been challenged to keep up with our social development. Chapter 2 offers a simplified but thorough discussion of the process of eyesight and the components of the visual system. The level of discussion is such that the health and safety professional will feel confident in learning how the eyes work and why subsequent recommendations are justified.

Next comes a discussion of the technology behind computer displays. Because the images created on a monitor differ from standard ink-on-paper, the eyes adjust to the image differently. An explanation of the terminology and image generation for the older cathode-ray tube (CRT) and the newer liquid crystal display (LCD) technologies are discussed.

The next chapters discuss the environmental issues surrounding eye symptoms and vision in the workplace. It covers lighting, glare, monitor position, viewing distances, and other issues in detail.

The American Optometric Association has defined computer vision syndrome (CVS) as "that complex of eye and vision problems related to near work that are experienced during or related to computer use." A complete discussion of the signs and symptoms of this condition is detailed and reviewed.

Following this is a discussion of lighting issues surrounding display use in the workplace. One of the major differences between viewing a display screen and viewing printed matter is that displays are self-illuminated, whereas paper requires external illumination. We explore the details of the quality of light and how to properly light a workplace so that all areas are clear and comfortable. A section on glare in the workplace is also included to clarify the role of anti-glare filters for displays.

Because the visual system is integral with body posture, we also include a section on general ergonomic principles. We tie in these general ergonomic concepts with the impact they have on the vision of computer users and show how they depend on each other.

The next chapter discusses how vision examinations differ for computer users as opposed to more traditional examinations. This is meant to inform the health and safety professional as to what information is critical to describe to the doctor. A discussion of "computer glasses" and how they are to be used in the workplace is included.

In addition to computer use, the next chapter discusses eye safety in industrial settings. This area not only covers safety glasses but also includes government standards, types of equipment, visual considerations, contact lenses, and more.

While not specifically involved with current office ergonomic consider-ations, the effect of computer use on children is also pertinent to this dis-cussion. A recent survey indicates that about 80% of children from the ages of 8 to 18 use computers on a regular basis. In addition, software makers now target their products for children as young as 18 months old! The future workforce is being created, and problems experienced while a young person will often carry over to productivity and performance in the workplace.

No discussion of ergonomics can be complete without including the eco-nomic impact of such programs in the workplace. Ergonomic considerations are often limited by the economics of a particular company. The book con-cludes with a discussion of these closely related issues.

The appendices include a computer vision questionnaire, an occupational vision questionnaire, resources for blind and visually impaired employees, a seal-of-approval list for antiglare filters from the American Optometric Association, a list of ergonomic accessories from various companies, and additional resources.

This book is a compilation of contributions from some of the best minds in the ergonomics community. While it is impossible to single out the best in any field, I feel confident that these professionals have significant contri-butions to make in the area of visual ergonomics. Following the Introduction is a roster of the contributors and short biographies noting their accomplish-ments.

The Editor

Jeffrey R. Anshel, B.S., O.D.

Dr. Jeffrey Anshel is a 1975 graduate of the Illinois College of Optometry. He served as a lieutenant in the U.S. Navy from 1975 to 1977 in San Diego, where he established the Navy's first vision therapy center. He has written numerous articles regarding nutritional influences on vision, stress factors that affect visual performance, and computer vision concerns.

In 1990, Dr. Anshel published his first book titled *Healthy Eyes, Better Vision*, a layman's reference book containing useful information and practical advice regarding vision care. His second book, *Visual Ergonomics in the Workplace*, published by Taylor & Francis, offers scientific and practical information about the interaction between computers and the visual system. It is a comprehensive guide to the role of vision in the workplace. *Smart Medicine For Your Eyes*, Dr. Anshel's third book, is a resource of remedies using conventional, nutritional, and homeopathic eye treatments.

Dr. Anshel is the principal of Corporate Vision Consulting, where he addresses the issues surrounding visual demands while working with computers. His work includes a course for eyecare professionals through which he educates doctors on computer vision syndrome and a course on dry eye syndrome. He also offers corporations on-site consultations and seminars related to visual stress in the workplace. Dr. Anshel is an assistant professor at the Southern California College of Optometry in Fullerton, California, and currently maintains a full-service practice in Carlsbad, California.

Contributors

Herb Berkwits, M.E.E.

For more than 30 years, Herb Berkwits has been involved in the design, marketing, and sales of all types and sizes of displays, from half-inch LCDs to huge stadium scoreboards. Originally hired as a display design engineer by Hughes Aircraft Company, he has more recently held management positions with leading display companies such as Mitsubishi and ViewSonic. Mr. Berkwits is currently the Senior Product Manager for Quest International, a distributor of high-performance LCD monitors for medical imaging. Mr. Berkwits holds a Bachelor's and a Master's Degree in Electrical Engineering from Cornell University.

James Sheedy, O.D., Ph.D.

Dr. Sheedy is an associate professor of optometry at The Ohio State University College of Optometry. He previously served as a clinical professor at the University of California at Berkeley School of Optometry, where he founded the first VDT Eye Clinic in 1985. He is widely recognized as the pre-eminent scientific and clinical expert on vision issues in the workplace — especially among computer users. He has been a public spokesperson on many eye-related issues, has appeared on several radio and television programs, and has been quoted in numerous publications including three times in *The Wall Street Journal* (once on the front page).

He is active in the American Optometric Association and the American Academy of Optometry, of which he is a fellow and a diplomate. He has also been active in the ophthalmic industry and has participated in the development of numerous standards and regulations, including ANSI, ISO, OSHA, and for state legislatures. He received the Distinguished Service Award from Prevent Blindness America for his work with ultraviolet protection and for coordinating the efforts of the American Optometric Association and the American Academy of Ophthalmology on this issue.

Dr. Sheedy has performed research into various areas of visual performance and visual symptoms, and has been recognized with several research awards, including twice receiving the Garland Clay Award for the best clinical research published in the journal of the American Academy of Optometry. He has also received the William Feinbloom Award from the

American Academy of Optometry for his contributions to vision care. He has more than 100 published articles and gives numerous lectures to both professional and lay groups. Currently, he continues his research and clinical work at his OSU Vision Ergonomics Research Laboratory.

Sharon M. Middendorf

Sharon M. Middendorf, senior technical marketing specialist in 3M's Optical Systems Division, manages the division's technical marketing, regulatory, and human factors applications and affiliations. She has degrees in history and physics and serves as a corporation expert on visual ergonomics and the computing environment. She served for five years on the International Standards Organization (ISO) working group for electronic display ergonomics and chaired the subcommittee for the introduction and scope of a new electronic display measurement consolidation standard.

Sharon has been a consultant for many different companies, including the New York Metropolitan Opera, ErgoNorms Compliance Center, Cornell University Human Factors Laboratory, and TÜV Rheinland Product Service. She has presented on "Vision and the Computing Environment" to Wells Fargo Bank, *La Opinion* newspaper, and ergonomic assessment teams within 3M. In addition to being a consultant, she holds many professional memberships, including the International Association of Privacy Professionals, the Human Factors and Ergonomics Society (HFES), the Computer Security Institute, the Society for Information Display, and the Standards Engineering Society.

Carolyn M. Sommerich, Ph.D.

Dr. Sommerich is an associate professor in the Department of Industrial, Welding & Systems Engineering at The Ohio State University and holds an adjunct appointment in the Department of Industrial Engineering at North Carolina State University. Her research focus is ergonomics and occupational biomechanics, with special interests in the upper body, upper extremities, and office ergonomics. She has received funding for research addressing biomechanical effects of computer monitor placement and keyboard design and use, and ergonomic aspects of portable computer use, as well as the study of risk factors for upper extremity musculoskeletal disorders in the furniture manufacturing industry and in agricultural work. She is the author of papers on a diverse range of ergonomics issues, including work-related musculoskeletal disorders of the shoulder, assessment of carpal tunnel pressure during keyboarding, and changes in patterns of trunk muscle activity in response to lifting task requirements.

Dr. Sommerich serves as a member of the editorial boards of the *Journal of Electromyography and Kinesiology* and *International Journal of Industrial Ergonomics*, and is an occasional reviewer for several peer-reviewed journals, including *Human Factors*, *Applied Ergonomics*, and *American Journal of Industrial Medicine*. She is the past chair of the Ergonomics Committee of the American Industrial Hygiene Association and is currently serving the Human Factors and Ergonomics Society as an at-large member of its Executive Council. She is also the faculty advisor to OSU's student chapter of HFES. She teaches courses at the graduate level in occupational biomechanics, upper extremity biomechanics, musculoskeletal mechanics, and user-centered design. She also teaches undergraduate courses in work analysis and design, ergonomics, and engineering economics. She graduated summa cum laude from the University of Cincinnati, with a B.S.M.E., and earned her M.S. and Ph.D. from The Ohio State University.

Stephen L. Glasser, O.D., FAAO

Dr. Glasser did his professional studies at the Pennsylvania College of Optometry, after completing undergraduate studies at The Ohio State University. Having practiced in Washington, DC, since 1976, Dr. Glasser's expertise has been sought by both television and print media. In addition, he has been recognized by his profession as practicing the highest standards of excellence — by being named as a fellow of the American Academy of Optometry, by being named one of the nation's "Best and Brightest" in the eye care field by *20/20 Magazine*, and by being named Optometrist of the Year by the Optometric Society of the District of Columbia for 1995.

Dr. Glasser lectures regularly on and is a consultant in the field of computer ergonomics. His presentations have taken him from Alaska to Florida, speaking to doctors, professional organizations, and office staffs alike. His consulting work has included work with law firms, media groups, governmental agencies, and international corporations. Dr. Glasser is in private practice in Washington, D.C.

Bernard R. Blais, M.D., FACOEM, FAAO, FACS

Dr. Blais is Clinical Professor of Ophthalmology at Albany Medical College, Albany, New York. He is co-chair of the ACOEM Sensory Perception Committee and serves on the Council on Scientific Affairs. He is board certified in ophthalmology.

He served for 30 years as a commissioned officer in the United States Navy, during which time, approximately 20 years, he was trained and subsequently trainer, as chairman of two ophthalmology departments at Naval Hospital Philadelphia and Naval Medical Center Bethesda, Maryland. In the subsequent 10 years, he was the Force Medical Officer of the Military Sealift Command (corporate medical director), Head of the Surface/Sealift Operational Division at Bureau of Medicine and Surgery, U.S. Navy.

From 1988 to 1996, he was Regional Medical Director, Lockheed-Martin Corporation (formerly General Electric Company) Knolls Atomic Power Laboratory (KAPL, Inc.), Schenectady, New York. This facility is a research development and training laboratory operated by Lockheed-Martin as a contractor for the Department of Energy (DOE) and the U.S. Navy–Naval Reactors Program. KAPL, Inc. has approximately 3,000 employees and 4,000 active duty personnel. The Medical Director was responsible for three sites at KAPL, Inc.: Knolls Site, Schenectady, New York; Kesselring Site, Saratoga Springs, New York; and Windsor Site in Windsor, Connecticut.

As president of Blais Consulting Ltd. in Clifton Park, New York, since July 1996, he is a consultant specializing in occupational ophthalmology. The goal is to organize and bring together information regarding eyes in the workplace. His combined years in ophthalmology and occupational medicine in the Navy provided him with expertise in occupational safety, eye care in the workplace, occupational visual standards, and visual ergonomics for the workplace.

Alan Hedge, Ph.D.

Dr. Hedge is a professor in the Department of Design and Environmental Analysis, Cornell University, where, since 1987, he has directed the Human Factors and Ergonomics teaching and research programs. Prior to that, for more than 10 years he ran the Graduate Program in Applied Psychology and Ergonomics at Aston University, Birmingham, U.K. From 1990 to 1993, he was also an Honorary Research Fellow at the Institute of Occupational Health, University of Birmingham, U.K. He is a fellow of the Human Factors and Ergonomics Society, a fellow of the Ergonomics Society (UK) and a Certified Professional Ergonomist. He received the 2003 Alexander J. Williams Jr. Design Award from the Human Factors and Ergonomics Society.

His research and teaching activities have focused on issues of design and workplace ergonomics as these affect the health, comfort, and productivity of workers. His research themes include workstation design and carpal tunnel syndrome risk factors for workers, alternative keyboard and input system designs, the performance and health effects of postural strain, and the health and comfort impacts of various environmental stressors, such as the effects of indoor air quality on sick building syndrome complaints among office workers, and the effects of office lighting on eyestrain problems among computer workers. He has co-edited the *Handbook of Human Factors and*

Ergonomics Methods, co-authored *Keeping Buildings Healthy: How to Monitor and Prevent Indoor Environmental Problems*, and published 30 chapters and more than 160 articles on these topics in the ergonomics and related journals.

Maurice Oxenburgh, B.Sc., Ph.D., FESA

Dr. Oxenburgh graduated from the University of New South Wales with a doctorate in biochemistry but, for the past quarter of a century, has worked in occupational health and safety, where his principal interests have been in occupational hygiene and ergonomics. In March 2000, he gave evidence in Washington, D.C., to support OSHA's proposed Ergonomics Standard.

While working in industry, Dr. Oxenburgh realized that, although managers wanted efficient workplaces, they saw safety as a cost. His experience showed otherwise, and he has taken it as an article of faith that a safe workplace is more effective, efficient, and productive than one that is not safe.

Dr Oxenburgh is presently ensconced as Emeritus Research Scholar at the National Institute for Working Life (Sweden), continuing his work on developing methods for measuring worker safety and productivity. He is a fellow of the Ergonomics Society of Australia.

Pepe Marlow, B.App.Sc., M.Com., MHFESA

Pepe Marlow has worked for 20 years in occupational health and safety where her principal interest has been in ergonomics. Early on in her career she experienced frustration in assisting workplaces to see the benefits of ergonomics and so went on to study economics, graduating from the University of New South Wales with a master's degree in commerce.

In 1997, Pepe prepared "Estimation of the regulatory impact of the national standard for manual handling component of the proposed consolidated OHS regulation" for WorkCover NSW, Australia. She developed a cost-benefit analysis of the impact of this standard based on available data and estimates for missing data.

Since that time, she has worked extensively with Maurice Oxenburgh, writing several publications showing how to calculate the cost benefit of occupational health and safety, as well as presenting at conferences and running workshops on the same subject.

Pepe is presently working as an occupational health and safety consultant, continuing her focus on assisting workplaces to see the benefits that come from improved ergonomics.

Introduction

"Seeing is believing"

"An eye for an eye"

"In the blink of an eye"

"I see what you mean"

Many of our oldest and wisest sayings deal with the eyes. That's probably because vision is our primary connection with the world. We use our eyes to interact with our environment in more than a million ways every second. The eyes really are an extension of the brain and a direct link between our environment and our minds. More than 80% of our learning comes from our vision, which indicates how important our sense of sight is in our daily lives.

The process of vision begins with visible light — a portion of the radiation spectrum that stimulates the nerve endings in the retina. The eyes can sense about 10 million gradations of light and about 7 million different shades of color. The retina is about the size of a postage stamp and is made up of about 130 million light-sensitive cells. It captures light and transforms it into nerve impulses, and it can form, dissolve, and create a new image every tenth of a second.

The eyes are truly the windows to our world and to our soul. Because of their connection to the brain, they influence most of our cognitive thought processes. When the computer was first developed in the late 1940s, it was most often compared to the brain — with a network of interconnections and a sense of logical "thinking." Even today, we tend to think that the computer is highly sophisticated and able to react as quickly and accurately as the human brain. And the way we primarily interact with the computer is through our eyes (the visual display).

The connection between the visual display and the eye is a natural one. The computer generates and organizes information for our needs and displays that information on the screen. We then capture that information with our eyes. You might think of the eyes as the connection between the two "brains" we use. In order to maintain that link, our visual system might make certain adaptations to ease the flow of information. These adaptations can often lead to other physical complications. Therefore, we should take care of our eyes to ensure that our computer viewing habits, viewing environment, and visual condition are all considered wherever we use the computer.

Using a computer is a twenty-first century necessity. The computer has surpassed the telephone as the number one essential office tool. Yet one significant difference remains between the telephone and the computer, and it involves vision. While you don't really have to see a telephone to use it, it's a very different story when it comes to computer use.

If you ask most people about their computer, they'll actually be thinking about the monitor or visual display. The main interaction people have with their computers is through their eyes, and statistics demonstrate the effects of this. A recent survey of computer users indicated that eyestrain is the main complaint of more than 80% of them. While carpal tunnel syndrome has become a common malady for many computer users, more people actually suffer from computer vision syndrome, or CVS. The American Optometric Association has designated CVS as the "complex of eye and vision problems related to near work that are experienced during or related to computer use." Much of the text herein is dedicated to defining and resolving this condition.

Because computer use is so very different from viewing paper-based tasks, our eyes have to make an adjustment in the way we see. As adaptable as we humans are, our eyes will most likely adapt to this new viewing situation, but not without the stress and strain that comes with a new viewing modality. It is the purpose of this book to review the research and concepts about vision as related to computer use, and to assist in making this new viewing situation as comfortable as possible.

It is hoped that this book serves as a cornerstone for a good understanding of the role vision plays in the lives of employees in the workplace. I have brought together some of the most revered experts in their respective fields to offer the most recent research and quality information available.

The efficiency with which we see relates directly to how efficiently and safely we perform on the job. We spend almost one third of our lives working and our eyes are the source of our most important sense. It is my hope that they work well throughout an entire lifetime.

1

Windows to the World

Jeffrey Anshel

CONTENTS

The eyes are simple tools designed to catch light. However, the method by which they gather, filter and guide the light, as well as the way in which our brains process the information received by the eyes, makes for the wonder of vision. In interacting with our environment, there is little to compare with the contribution of the eyes. The way we use our eyes and visual systems dictates how well we survive in our environment. In order to understand how the eyes and visual system are designed to work, we might first look at our development from a historical perspective — both physically and socially.

Our Ancestral Eyes

The current species of man, *Homo sapiens*, first appeared about 40,000 years ago. Our ancestors were designed to survive in a difficult and challenging environment. Finding food, shelter, protection, and survival were the first priorities, while the "comforts" of clothing and amenities were secondary. Their bodies developed to support their needs: flexibility, agility, and strength. And if successful, they lived to the ripe old age of 25 to 30 years, according to most authorities.

Likewise, the eyes of our ancestors were designed for a similar type of survival. They were situated in a frontal position so the visual fields could overlap and work together, creating the sense of stereoscopic vision — the ability to perceive depth. They are near the top of the body so as to afford the longest range of sight. Since eyes were used mostly during the daytime, daytime vision was keen; night vision was adequate but secondary. The eyes were also developed for motility — moving in many directions, in conjunction with head movements, to be able to view a wide radius of the horizon.

This "hunter/gatherer" type of visual system is the same one we are using today. We now, however, view our world for about 16 hours a day, with much of that in artificial light and in an environment that is mostly within arm's reach. We read small items of text in various lighting situations for hours on end and struggle to meet deadlines that are imposed upon us. During much of the year, our eyes are exposed to very little daylight for any extended period of time. We ask our eyes and visual system to adapt to these adverse conditions and they must make the necessary adaptations to assure our survival. These changes are slow to develop and not always successful for what we need to accomplish. Often, sacrifices are made in one area of vision for the sake of seeing better in other situations.

The Information Age

Our success as humans developed mostly because of our ability to provide for ourselves. We learned how to hunt and to outsmart our predators. We also learned how to plant food and combine our hunting with agricultural skills so as to proliferate. Until the late nineteenth century, we were largely an agricultural society that used these skills for survival. Our eyes maintained their ability to see clearly at distances during daylight hours with occasional near viewing.

The transformation in our visual development began in the late 1870s with the invention of the light bulb. With this new technology, we were able to extend our comfortable viewing into the nighttime hours. Other developments and technological advances led to the start of the Industrial Age, during which machines were developed to help us in our daily living. The automobile and the airplane are prime examples of machines that have had a major impact on our society. Driving vision consists of a combination of distance and intermediate viewing, with the distance being most critical. Along with this development came the need for closer inspection of machine parts, dials, and other mechanical devices. Near-point viewing was a critical task and the success of these and other machines depended upon it. The success of employees working in this situation is directly related to how efficiently they use their eyes. Poor vision reduces a worker's performance and productivity, as well as increasing the risk of having an accident on the job.

A significant part of this development was a parallel development in the electronics field that assisted in the function of the machines. About midway through the twentieth century, the computer was developed and our society once again began to shift. Because of its unique ability to do basic arithmetic and other numerical calculations, the computer gradually became (and continues to become) an integral part of our newly dawning Information Age. Although it wasn't obvious at first, the visual requirements for computing are different from what is required for viewing other types of mechanical equipment. Working with a self-illuminated video display terminal (VDT) screen at an awkward angle of view and unique working distance is yet another adaptation our visual system has had to make. It is noteworthy that this last transformation occurred less than 100 years from the previous shift, which is extremely rapid in historical terms.

An Eye on the Future

As computer viewing becomes more commonplace and becomes our standard of operation, the problems that arise are likely to be compounded. While only 10% of the workforce was using computers for their daily activities in 1980, that percentage has climbed to more than 80% today and is expected to reach the 185 million mark in the next few years. Computers are getting faster and "smarter," the technology of display design and quality is improving, and they are becoming more affordable. Yet, there are still major considerations to address. In 1991, a Lou Harris poll cited computer-related eyestrain as the number one office health complaint in the United States. That same year, a study by the National Institute for Occupational Safety and Health (NIOSH) indicated that 88% of the 66 million people who work at computers for more than three hours a day, nearly 60 million, were suffering from symptoms of eyestrain. As recently as 2004, a survey of more than 1000 consumers indicated that more than 61% were concerned about vision problems resulting from prolonged computer use. More than 60% of respondents also believe that these problems will worsen in the future and that they could affect routine activities.

Although problems with computer eyestrain outstripped carpal tunnel syndrome and other more high-profile office health complaints more than a decade ago, the size of this epidemic has not received the attention it warrants. The reason is that a key cause of computer eyestrain has not been well understood. Eye problems are most often painless and slow to develop, thus they are often misdiagnosed as other conditions, such as migraine headaches or tiredness.

An additional concern is the potential for vision and other physical problems in children, who are growing up using this new technology on a full-time basis. Children's computer-using habits are not yet being addressed in any significant way. Ergonomic furniture, monitor placement, mouse dimensions, proper lighting, body posturing, and many other factors have yet to be considered. Add to this equation the amount of time children spend looking at computer-generated games and schoolwork and the potential for serious complications is looming.

In addition, the role of eye-care practitioners will also shift as the viewing situations of their patients change. The role of eye care providers must keep up with the demands of their patients. Doctors must analyze problems that arise due to the interaction of workers/patients with their environments, be called on to design optimal viewing environments, and evaluate those environments to improve visual performance. This may transform the way routine eye examinations are performed.

Our "future vision" may once again be one of adaptation. However, several considerations must be addressed and, as of this writing, it appears that we don't even have all of the questions, much less the answers we require. It is likely that just as we now routinely accept that sunglasses are appropriate for a sunny day, we may need to accept that computer-viewing glasses are just as appropriate. No matter what type of input device is found to make our entries easier (e.g., voice activation), the output of computers will always involve the visual system. Our eyes will need to learn to adapt to these stressful viewing situations, but we must know how we can help ease that transition.

2

The Eyes and Visual System

Jeffrey Anshel

CONTENTS

Eyeball Basics

This book is not meant to be a technical medical synopsis of the anatomy and physiology of the human visual system. However, you should know some basic information about how the eye is put together and how it works in order to have some background with which to make intelligent decisions regarding vision requirements in the workplace. We'll start with some basic eye anatomy so that you know what is what and where it is. Then, you can understand how the parts work together to create this fascinating organ.

The eyeball is basically that — a ball (Figure 2.1). Its diameter is roughly an inch, and it's about three inches in circumference. The part of the eye that is visible to the world — between the eyelids — is actually only one sixth of the eye's total surface area. The remaining five sixths of the eyeball is hidden behind the eyelids. The outer surface of the eye is divided into two parts: the sclera (SKLER-ah), the white part that is the outer covering of the eye, and the cornea (KOR-nee-ah), the transparent membrane in front of the eye. The cornea, which is steeper in curvature than the sclera, may be difficult

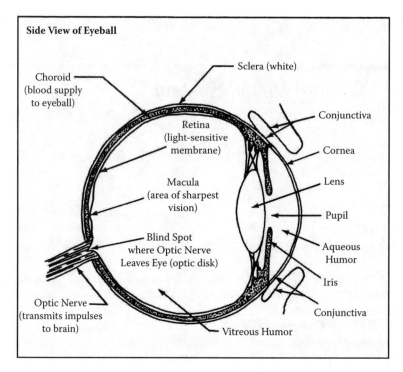

Side View of Eyeball

Choroid
(blood supply
to eyeball)

Sclera (white)

Retina
(light-sensitive
membrane)

Conjunctiva

Cornea

Macula
(area of sharpest
vision)

Lens

Pupil

Blind Spot
where Optic Nerve
Leaves Eye (optic disk)

Aqueous
Humor

Iris

Optic Nerve
(transmits impulses
to brain)

Conjunctiva

Vitreous Humor

FIGURE 2.1
Side view of an eyeball.

to see because it is transparent and the colored iris (EYE-ris) is behind it. You can see the cornea most easily if you look at a friend's eye from the side. The sclera is made of tough fibers, which allow it to perform its function as the supporting structure for the contents of the eyeball. It has a white appearance because the fibers are light in color and because there are very few blood vessels in it.

Just inside the sclera and covering most of the same area is the choroid (KOH-royd), which is the main blood supply to the inner eyeball. And just inside the choroid is the retina (RET-in-ah), the nerve membrane that receives the light. In addition to the blood vessels of the choroid, there are also blood vessels that enter the eye through the optic nerve and lie on the front surface of the retina. They supply nutrition to the retina and other structures inside the eye. These parts all seem to be very basic when you think of what an eye must do. The eye needs protection and support (provided by the sclera), a blood supply (provided by the choroid and through the optic nerve) and a mechanism for seeing (provided by the retina and optic nerve).

As you look at an eye, the first thing you'll notice is the colored iris. If you look closely at an eye, you'll see that the iris is actually enclosed in what's known as a chamber, which is a medical term for a closed space. The iris is also surrounded by a watery fluid called the aqueous (AY-kwee-us) humor or aqueous fluid. "Humor" doesn't have anything to do with being funny;

it's just the Latin word for fluid. Just behind the iris is the crystalline lens, which provides the focusing part of the vision process. The lens is transparent and can't really be seen from the outside unless special equipment is used. Behind it, and filling the main chamber within the eye, is the vitreous (VIT-tree-us) humor. The vitreous humor is more gel-like and less watery than the aqueous humor and helps support the retina and other structures.

How the Eye Works

Let's look at the visual process by starting at the beginning. Light enters the eye by passing through the cornea, the aqueous humor and the pupil; is focused by the lens; and then goes through the vitreous humor and onto the retina. It was noted that the retina is actually an extension of the brain. That's right! The nerve fibers from the retina form the optic nerves, which go directly into the brain (Figure 2.2).

The light that strikes the retina first stimulates chemical changes in the light-sensitive cells of the retina, known as the photoreceptors. There are actually two kinds of photoreceptors: The rods, which are long, slender cells, respond to light or dark stimuli and are important to our night vision; the cones, which are cone-shaped, respond to color stimuli and therefore are also called color receptors. There are about 17 times as many rods as there are cones — about 120 million rods and 7 million cones in the retina of each

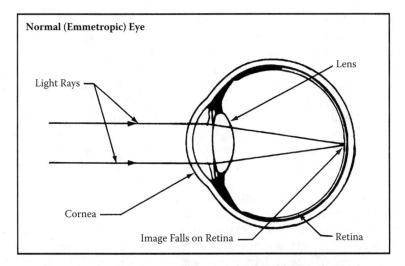

FIGURE 2.2
In the normal eye, an image falls exactly on the retina. The shape of the eyeball and cornea are normal, and the eye's lens has normal flexibility and focusing ability.

eye. These rods and cones interconnect and converge to form a network of about 1 million nerve fibers that make up each optic nerve.

When light strikes the rods and cones, they convert the light energy to nerve energy; we'll call this nerve energy a visual impulse. This impulse travels out of the eye into the brain via the optic nerve at a speed of 423 miles per hour. It first reaches the middle of the brain where a pair of "relay stations" combines the visual information it is carrying with other sensory information. The impulse then travels to the very back part of the brain, the visual cortex. It is here that the brain interprets the shapes of objects and the spatial organization of a scene and recognizes visual patterns as belonging to a known object — for example, it recognizes that a flower is a flower. Further visual processing is done at the sides of the brain, known as the temporal lobes. Once the brain has interpreted vital information about something the eyes have "seen," it instantaneously transfers this information to many areas of the brain. For example, if the information is that a car is moving toward you, it is relayed to the motor cortex, which is the area that controls movement and enables you to get out of the way.

So, vision is really a process that uses the eyeball to receive images (commonly called eyesight) and the brain interpreting the signals from the eye (the visual process).

Refractive Errors

The process I've just described is how the normal eye and visual system function when they work perfectly well. This condition of the optically normal eye is called emmetropia (em-e-TROH-pee-ah). Unfortunately, this isn't always the case. Very often there is something that goes wrong and the visual process is disrupted. About 50% of the adults in the United States have difficulty seeing clearly at a distance and about 60% have difficulty seeing near with no corrective lenses. One of the more common problems is the misfocusing of the light as it is directed onto the retina. The light can focus too soon, too late, or be distorted. Because the bending of light is technically called "refraction," the misfocusing of light in the eye is called a "refractive error."

First, let's clarify these terms. Nearsightedness, also called myopia (my-OH-pee-ah), means having good near vision but poor distance vision. For the myopic person, a distant image (an image at least 20 feet away, so that the eye's lens is as relaxed as it can be) falls in front of the retina and looks blurred (Figure 2.3). Nearsightedness results when an eye is too long, when the cornea is too steeply curved, when the eye's lens is unable to relax enough to provide accurate distance vision, or from some combination of these and other factors.

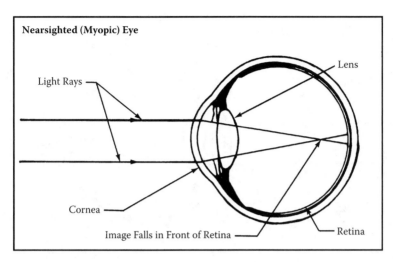

FIGURE 2.3
In the nearsighted eye, the image falls in front of the retina when the lens is in its' relaxed state, viewing an object that is at least 20 feet away. The image is blurred.

Farsightedness, also called hyperopia (hy-per-OH-pee-ah), is not exactly the opposite of myopia. For the hyperopic person, an object that is 20 feet or more away (so that the lens is relaxed) is directed past the retina, so that it looks blurred because it hasn't yet focused (Figure 2.4). Farsightedness results when an eye is too short or the cornea too flat, or from some combination of these and other factors. The main difference between these two conditions is that they eye can increase its focal power (to some degree) to compensate for farsightedness, whereas it can't reduce its power to compensate for nearsightedness.

Theoretically, the surface of the cornea should be almost spherical in shape, like the surface of a ball, so that when light passes through it, it can be focused at a single point. However, nature isn't always perfect, and the cornea is often "warped" so that it more closely resembles a barrel than a ball. The lens too can be irregular in shape. These distortions can be significant enough so that the light that passes through the cornea and lens in the vertical orientation will focus at a different spot from the light that passes through in the horizontal orientation. Now you have two points of focus with a blur between them. This is known as astigmatism (a-STIG-ma-tism) (Figure 2.5).

If the difference between these two points of focus is great enough, the eye will strain trying to decide which point of focus it should use. You might then develop occasional blurring of vision, tiring, or possibly headaches. Astigmatism in small amounts is very common and not of great concern. But, about 23 million Americans have a significant amount of astigmatism that requires correction. Glasses correct astigmatism by having curvatures that compensate for the curvature of the eye. This is a simple optical correction, and the glasses will not change the amount of astigmatism; that is, they won't "cure" the problem.

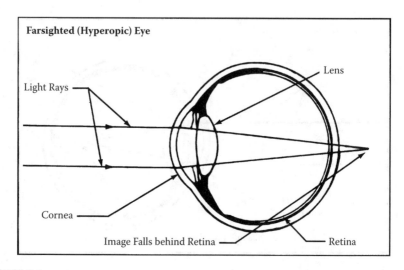

FIGURE 2.4
In the farsighted eye, the image falls behind the retina when the lens is in its relaxed state, viewing an object that is at least 20 feet away. The image is blurred.

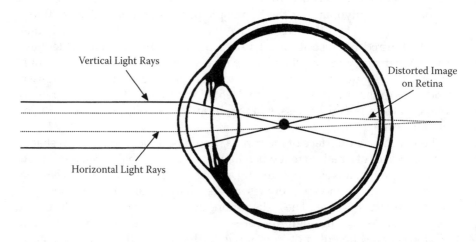

FIGURE 2.5
In astigmatism, the image that enters the eye is distorted (usually by the cornea) and does not have a single point of focus.

Seeing Clearly Now

Recall the last time you visited your eye doctor's office. You probably got a full examination, had what seemed like a hundred different tests, and you asked: "How are my eyes?" The answer could have been: "You have 20/20 vision!" You then walked out of the office satisfied that your eyes were in good shape. But are they? What does 20/20 refer to and what does it mean?

These numbers are really just a notation that relates to the resolving power of the eye. Resolving power means how sharp your sight is, which we can define as your ability to distinguish two points from each other and not see them as just one point. If your vision is 20/20, it means that you're seeing at 20 feet what the optically normal eye can see at 20 feet — that is, that your eyes can distinguish one point from another on a specific line from a standard eye chart placed 20 feet away. The chart is called a Snellen chart. If your vision is, let's say, 20/40, it means that you can see at 20 feet what the normal eye can see at 40 feet (you have to be closer). And, if your vision is 20/100, you must be at 20 feet while the normal eye can be 100 feet away and see the same thing as clearly. In short, the larger the bottom number is, the poorer your resolving power, which is also known as your visual acuity. Visual acuity is measured for distance and near vision. So now you know that 20/20 is something like a grading of eyesight.

Binocular Vision

Seeing a clear 20/20 is certainly a good indication that your eyes might be doing a good job. However, sharp eyesight is just one of the functions that your eyes perform. Since we have two eyes, we must make sure that they are working in harmony with each other. One of the most fascinating abilities of the visual system is to take images from two eyes and put them together into just one picture. You don't normally see two images, so the idea might sound strange, but double vision can occur and is one of the most dangerous manifestations of vision problems. Imagine seeing two cars coming at you as you drive down the road!

Here's how the brain keeps us from going off the road. Let's assume that you have two eyes and they are both working about equally well. As you look at just one object, each eye receives an image of that object. Both of these images are transmitted back to your brain, but they are then fused together by the brain into one image. In order for that to happen, both eyes must be pointed at the same object, and the images have to be approximately equal in size and clarity.

Now, if one eye does not aim at the same spot as the other, each eye will be looking at a different object, and the two images won't match up. When the images are transmitted back to your brain, they will stimulate two different groups of brain cells, and you will experience two images: seeing double. After a short time, your brain will decide to turn off, or suppress, the picture from the eye that is pointed in the wrong direction so that you can see one image again. This suppression is necessary for our visual survival, but it is not the way we were made to see.

This suppression of an image is the brain's way to make our daily tasks easy and comfortable in stressful situations. Thus, you might think that suppression of an image is devastating but it actually works pretty well. What is more serious, however, is when there is a competition between the eyes and they are struggling to work together. This problem is much more common than the suppression problem. It is this competition that causes the person to struggle with reading tasks and can lead to poor reading comprehension and job performance. Adequate binocular function is important to successful work related tasks.

Visual Skills for Computer Users

Let's take a look at the task of viewing a computer display and note the various visual skills that are required to do it comfortably and efficiently.

First, there is visual acuity. If the letters viewed on the screen are not clear, then the user cannot perform the task effectively. Blurred letters at the screen distance can be caused by a number of conditions that we will discuss shortly. For now, just understand that clarity, without excess effort, is essential to proper computer use. Next, there is accommodation. Accommodation is the act of refocusing the light when viewing a near object as opposed to viewing a distant object. This entails using the crystalline lens (just behind the iris) to adjust its shape, which in turn alters its focusing power. There are many facets to evaluating accommodation but the two of significance here are the maximum ability and the flexibility. The maximum focusing ability determines whether the image can be brought into clear focus onto the retina; the flexibility determines whether it can be done easily and also reversed to regain distant vision with ease. Both of these factors must be mastered by the visual system of the computer user to ensure clear and comfortable viewing.

Binocular vision — the efficient use of both eyes together — is also necessary, but this might be subject to debate. It is true that many "one-eyed" people can use a computer with ease and comfort, so you might think that binocular vision is not important. However, remember that the suppression of one of the eyes' images is effective for our daily function but is not optimum. It is, again, the close competition between the two eyes that can lead to decreased performance if not coordinated with efficiency. Scanning and tracking, both eye movement skills, must also be performed smoothly for the user to make accurate visual moves. Scanning involves the eyes jumping over the image as a whole with the ability to perceive many images at once and then locate the one desired. Tracking is the type of movement that is used in reading, where small jumps are made at regular intervals so as to follow an orderly progression. The computer user must be able to perform these skills efficiently to keep from overusing and tiring the eye muscles.

Glare recovery is a significant factor in computer use because of the many sources of glare found in the workplace. This topic will be covered in much more detail later, but the eye's ability to recover from glare is normally determined by the function of the retina and other optical properties within the eye. Proper nutrition and eye health are critical factors in glare recovery abilities.

Hand–eye coordination is also a function that the user must master to effectively input data into a computer. Using the feedback from the visual system, keyboard entry will determine what the next entry is to be. Also, efficient mouse manipulation is determined by hand–eye coordination abilities.

Developing Myopia

The latest demographic figures show that 58% of the U.S. population as a whole wears some form of vision correction. And about 32% of them are nearsighted, or myopic. This should be a rather surprising statistic considering that less than 2% of the population is born nearsighted. There is still some controversy as to what is the exact cause of myopia, but new research is shedding some light on the subject (Zadnick et al., 1995).

It's been believed for a long time now that myopia is inherited, and we shouldn't overlook the contribution of a heredity factor. But, this is probably not the whole story because myopia is much more prevalent in people and societies where close work is a significant part of daily life. Studies have found, for example, that myopia is almost nonexistent in uneducated societies (such as early Eskimos or some African tribes) and that myopia increases in proportion to the amount of education in any given society (Young et al., 1969). In other words, the more reading and near-point work a society does, the higher the incidence of myopia.

In a similar vein, studies have been conducted with Navy submariners (Schwartz and Sandberg, 1954), who were submerged for months at a time, in a space where their maximum viewing distance is about eight feet. The studies showed an increase in myopia during these extended periods of confinement.

Dr. Francis Young of Washington University has done similar research with Rhesus monkeys (Young, 1963). He kept the monkeys in confined areas during various developmental periods of their early lives. His research showed that the shorter the maximum viewing distance and the longer the confinement, the more myopia the monkeys developed.

So what does this say about the way our eyes develop? As with any biological system, our visual system will change in response to stress. While reading printed text, your eyes are focused at a close distance — usually about 14 to 16 inches. The eye accomplishes this focusing through the process of accommodation. If this posture is maintained for long periods of time without a rest, the eyes slowly adapt to the position in order to reduce the stress on the muscles controlling each eye's lens. Once adapted, the eyes can see more clearly up close with less effort. It's as if the muscles get comfortably stuck in the near-focus position. To make matters worse, when the eye muscles work constantly to accommodate for near work, they cause some increased pressure to build up in the eye. Eventually, this pressure causes the eyeball itself to lengthen (which relieves the pressure), moving the retina farther back from the lens than it originally was.

So, what is the result of all this stress at the close working distance? Myopia. When the myopic eye relaxes the accommodation effort and attempts to refocus to a distant object, the image is blurred because it is over-focused too far forward of the retina. This process doesn't happen by just reading steadily for a night or two. It's a gradual adaptation that your eyes go through as they react to the strain of overwork.

As you might expect, myopia increases in children as they spend more and more of their time focused on near-vision activities. According to early statistical studies (Hirsch, 1952), about 1.6% of children entering school in the United States have some degree of myopia. That figure grows to 4.4% for 7- and 8-year-olds, 8.7% for 9- and 10-year-olds, 12.5% for 11- and 12-year-olds and 14.3% for 13- and 14-year-olds. We used to say that the progression (worsening) of myopia stabilized at maturity, about 21 years of age. However, over the past 15 or so years, eyecare professionals have seen more myopia progressing well into the late 20s or even 30s. The reason? We're not quite sure, but computers and their accompanying display screens are almost certainly to be considered one of the culprits.

While no research has shown that the display screens themselves have created more myopia in our society, my sense is that it is more likely caused by the amount of time we are spending viewing the computer display. Whereas we used to type a letter, go make a copy of it, write an envelope, go to the mailbox, etc., now we just do it all with the push of a button — while still looking at the same working distance: the computer screen!

References

Hirsch, M.J. Visual anomalies among children of grammar school age, *Archives of the American Academy of Optometry*, 23:11, 1952.

Schwartz, J. and Sandberg, N.E. Visual characteristics of submarine population, *Medical Research Laboratory*, US Navy Sub Base, North London, 13, 1954.

Young, F.A. et al. The transmission of refractive errors within Eskimo families, *Archives of the American Academy of Optometry*, 46:9, 1969.

Young, F.A. The effect of restricted visual space on refractive error on the young monkey's eyes, *Investigative Ophthalmology*, 2, 1963.

Zadnick, K. et al. Orinda longitudinal study of myopia, *Proceedings of the American Academy of Optometry*, Dec. 1995.

3

Electronic Visual Displays

Herb Berkwits

CONTENTS

It is somewhat ironic that the single component in one's computer system that makes the largest contribution to a satisfying and comfortable experience is the component that is usually thought about the least, i.e., the visual display. When we buy a computer, we discuss the processor speed, the available RAM, the size of the hard drive, etc., but rarely do we specify anything more than screen size when speaking of a display. To further the irony, the image that is produced by the latest Giga-whiz-bang processor, multi-Terabyte, shiny new computer typically reaches our eyes via a technology that is more than 100 years old — the cathode ray tube (CRT) monitor.

This chapter will discuss the available commercial display technologies, their strengths and weaknesses, what to look for and how to optimize the selected device.

The Cathode Ray Tube Display

The CRT is a light-emitting device. As previously mentioned, the CRT was first demonstrated more than 100 years ago. It is a fairly simple device to describe, but one requiring great precision to manufacture. The CRT consists of a glass bottle under a high vacuum with a layer of phosphorescent material at one end and an electron gun at the other. The electron gun creates a stream of electrons that are accelerated toward the phosphor by a very high voltage. When the electrons strike the phosphor, it glows at the point of impact. A coil of wire called the yoke is wrapped around the neck of the CRT. The yoke actually consists of a horizontal coil and a vertical coil, each of which generates a magnetic field when a voltage is applied. These fields deflect the beam of electrons both horizontally and vertically, thereby illuminating the entire screen rather than a pinpoint. To create an image, the electron beam is modulated (turned on and off) by the signal from the video card as it sweeps across the phosphor from left to right. When it reaches the right side of the tube, the beam is turned off or "blanked" and moved down one line and back to the left side. This process occurs repeatedly until the beam reaches the bottom right-hand side and is blanked and moved to the top left.

The number of addressable dots produced by the video card is called the horizontal resolution. The number of lines on the screen from top to bottom is called the vertical resolution. These are often referred to by the shorthand shown in Table 3.1.

IBM coined the original computer terms for the monochrome display adapter (MDA) and color graphics adapter (CGA) available with the early PCs. As the resolution and number of displayable colors increased, third-party display manufacturers coined new terms. While these terms were once useful, they have since lost any real meaning. Now they just refer to the various resolutions, as listed in Table 3.1. The "S" referred to super, "X" was extended, "U" was ultra, etc. With the new 16:9 screens, the terminology is just getting silly — QUXGAW, etc.

The previous discussion pertains to a monochrome or black-and-white CRT. Color CRTs are relative newcomers as they have only been around for about 60 years. Their construction is more complex, as color is achieved by

TABLE 3.1

Horizontal and Vertical Resolution

H Resolution (Dots)	V Resolution (Lines)	Computer Term
640	480	VGA
800	600	SVGA
1024	768	XGA
1280	1024	SXGA
1600	1200	UXGA

having three electron guns, each of which excites a phosphor that emits one of the primary colors, red, green, and blue, respectively. Phosphor dots or stripes for each of the primary colors are deposited on the CRT in groups of three called triads, and each triad is capable of displaying all colors from black to white by mixing different amounts of each color.

The Liquid Crystal Display

The liquid crystal display (LCD), or "flat panel" as it is sometimes called, is a totally different way of generating a computer display. Rather than being light emissive as is the CRT, the LCD is light transmissive. Each dot on the screen acts like an electrically controlled shutter that either blocks or passes a very high intensity backlight (or backlights) that is always on at full brightness.

Whereas the dots comprising the image of a CRT-based display vary in size depending upon the displayed resolution (if you display VGA resolution, the entire screen is lit with $640 \times 480 = 307,200$ dots while if you display UXGA, the screen is filled by $1600 \times 1200 = 1,920,000$ dots), an LCD panel has a fixed number of dots, called pixels or "picture elements." Each pixel is made up of three subpixels, a red, a green, and a blue. Since the backlight is white, the colors are achieved by means of tiny red, green, and blue filters.

Although the properties of a liquid crystal material were discovered in the late 1800s, it was not until 1968 that the first LCD display was demonstrated. Simply, light from the backlight is polarized, passed through the liquid crystal material (which twists the light 90 degrees) and passed through a second polarizer that is aligned with the first one. This results in a structure that blocks the backlight. The liquid crystal (LC) material has a unique property, however, that causes its molecules to line up with an applied voltage. The 90-degree twist goes to zero and the polarizer sandwich becomes transparent to the backlight. By applying more or less voltage, the light can be varied from zero (black) to 100% (white). Modern displays can make the transition from full off to full on in 256 steps, which in "digispeak" is 8 bits ($2^8 = 256$). Each pixel can display 256 shades each of red, green and blue for a total palette of $256 \times 256 \times 256 = 16.7$ million colors.

It is interesting that many monitor manufacturers will use that 16.7 million-color number very prominently in their advertising. However, in this book we are considering the eyes and visual system. Just how many colors does the human visual system perceive? Well, as near as we can tell (and there are no solid numbers here), the human visual system perceives from 7 to 8 million colors (in the most generous estimates). So, here we have a display that produces 16.7 million colors, but we can only see about half of those! For this reason, high-performance monochrome monitors used for medical imaging are often measured in "just noticeable differences," or JNDs.

As previously noted, the LCD has a fixed number of pixels that may be addressed by the video card regardless of the resolution being displayed. This is known as the "native resolution" of the panel. (Remember this — there will be a quiz.) Using the example of the UXGA display, there are 3 × 1,920,000 subpixels, or 5.76 million transistors controlling an equal number of dots on the screen.

While we're still discussing the "flat" panel, I'd like to mention the difference in terminology that I often hear. Many people refer to their "flat screen" display and really mean an LCD flat panel. The newer, professional-grade CRTs often have a flat piece of glass on their front surface, compared with the traditional convex glass of yesteryear. This is done to better control reflections and glare. So, the CRT is actually the display with a flat "screen" and the LCD is the flat "panel."

Getting the Image to the Display

To avoid the chaos that characterized the early days of computers, video card manufacturers and display manufacturers formed a standards committee called VESA. By specifying the type of signal, the voltages, the timing, and even the connector, modern monitors and modern computers almost always work nicely together. There is, however, a difference between the technology of a CRT and an LCD display that warrants driving them differently.

The CRT is basically an analog device. Data to be displayed starts at the computer in digital form and is converted to analog by a (I think you may be way ahead of me here) digital to analog converter (DAC). The CRT display uses these analog signals directly to drive the electron guns. The cable carries analog signals and this interface is often referred to as analog or VGA. Recall that VGA originally referred to "video graphic array," a video card that produced a resolution of 640 × 480 pixels. We have come a long way since the first VGA cards hit the market, yet the name lingers as a description of the connector, which is more correctly called 15-pin, high-density, D connector. (You now understand why people use VGA as shorthand.)

LCDs, however, are digital devices and appear to the computer as large arrays of memory. Since CRTs are still the dominant display technology, the LCD monitors are designed to work with the analog input and convert it to digital with its internal (this is getting easy) analog to digital converter (ADC). Since we start with digital data and end with digital data, would it not make sense to save two converters and keep everything digital? There is an industry standard called DVI (digital visual interface), which does just that. Better LCD monitors have both types of input, but the superior method of connecting an LCD monitor to your computer is DVI, if your display adapter supports it. All of the adjustments needed to get the best image when driving an LCD with an analog input are eliminated and the monitor simply becomes "plug and play."

Which Technology Is Superior?

Both LCD and CRT displays have advantages and disadvantages. It is up to the user to determine which is best for his or her application. The following are the major differences:

Size

The physical size of a CRT is considerably larger than an LCD display of the same screen size. Where LCD monitors remain thin as the screen area increases, the CRT grows in depth. A 21" CRT monitor might be more than 2 feet deep while a 21" LCD is only 3 or 4 inches. Thus, the LCD monitor can fit into spaces that the CRT cannot. Just think what your new SUV would look like if the movie screen in the back and the navigation system up front used CRT displays.

Furthermore, the specified viewable size of an LCD monitor and a CRT monitor are measured differently. Historically, the CRT is measured on a diagonal from edge to edge on the glass bottle even though it is incapable of creating an image at the extreme edges. Thus, the true viewable diagonal of a CRT is one to two inches less than the advertised size. LCD monitors, on the other hand, are specified by their true viewable diagonal measurement. In other words, a 21" CRT and a 20" LCD have the same viewable area. Advantage — LCD.

Power Consumption

LCD monitors typically use one third the power of a CRT monitor of similar screen size. As a result they generate less heat. This is usually trivial for a home computer, but for companies using hundreds of monitors in a single room (think stock brokerage or call centers), the energy savings from reduced power and reduced air conditioning load can be significant. Advantage — LCD

Viewing Angle

Older LCD monitors had very limited capability to display a good image when the viewer was not directly in front of the screen. The newer LCD displays are much better and sport viewing angles up to 170 degrees both vertically and horizontally. This measurement is somewhat misleading as it is taken where contrast ratio drops to 10:1 from 300:1 or more. Thus, the image at the extremes of the viewing angle is not nearly as good as the image seen directly in front of the display. CRT displays do not suffer any degradation at the viewing extremes. If your display will be used often for collaboration, CRT is your first choice. Advantage — CRT

Video Response Speed

This specification is the speed at which a display can turn a pixel from full black to full white and back to black. It is often quoted for LCDs but not for CRTs. Whereas an LCD display is considered fast (at this printing) if its response is 16 milliseconds (ms), a typical CRT has a response 50 times faster. Response speed is important if the image is dynamic, such as a movie or video game, as a slow panel leaves a trail or smear behind moving objects. It is much less a factor if the display is used for word processing or email.

One of the little secrets of the LCD manufacturers is that it often takes more time to transition between close shades of gray than it does to go from black to white to black. Thus, a single number cannot represent response speed faithfully. This is borne out by the observation that some 25ms panels exhibit less smearing than 16ms panels. Advantage — CRT

Eye Comfort

This can be very subjective, but the LCD exhibits no linearity or pincushion (straight lines looking curved) distortion and no flicker, all of which can contribute to computer vision syndrome or CVS (see next chapter). Furthermore, the LCD is always perfectly focused as long as it is set to display at its native resolution (I told you to remember this term). When displaying a non-native resolution, the LCD invokes a digital processor called a scaler to add enough pixels to fill the screen without distorting the image. This is a very complex procedure and the final result is a slightly softened image that many people find tiring. A good rule of thumb is to run an LCD monitor at its native resolution unless there is a compelling reason not to do so.

The electron beam in a CRT display is constantly scanning or drawing the image over and over. When it hits a specific spot on the screen, light is emitted, but as soon as the beam moves on, the spot starts to fade. It is critical that the beam scans all the points on the screen and returns to the first point in a short enough time that the eye does not perceive the dimming. The number of times an image is "painted" on the CRT is called the refresh rate or vertical sync frequency and it must be set to a value ≥75Hz to avoid flicker. Some people are hypersensitive to flicker and need an even higher refresh rate. The LCD display does not flicker by design. Advantage — LCD.

Cost

Although the cost of LCD monitors has plummeted in the last five years, the venerable CRT has come down in price almost equally as fast. Thus, an LCD monitor is still three to four times more expensive to purchase than a CRT display with the same screen size. This, however, does not tell the whole story. A display is considered to be at the end of its useful life when the luminance or brightness of the display is one half of the original luminance. Barring component failure, there are two aging mechanisms for a CRT — the electron gun develops an oxide coating and becomes less efficient, and the phosphor ages and emits less light for a given electron density. End of life for a CRT is 10,000 to 15,000 hours. The only aging mechanism for an LCD display is that the backlight(s) get dimmer. End of life for an LCD is ~50,000 hours with some new designs capable of up to 100,000 hours. Since the LCD will last anywhere from three to five times longer than a CRT, the total cost of ownership (TCO) is about equal.

It is worth noting that the use of a screen saver does *not* increase the life of an LCD monitor. Screen savers were designed to prevent a static image like a spreadsheet or word processing document from forming a permanent image, known as phosphor burn, when left on a CRT monitor screen for a long time. This is not a problem for the LCD monitor. Since the backlight of an LCD monitor is always on at its maximum luminance, the only way to increase the life of the display is to turn the backlight off when the display is not in use. This can be accomplished very simply by turning on the power management function in the operating system. Not only does this save power, it also increases the useful lifetime of the display. Advantage — tie

How to Buy

There are several specifications that are published for CRT and LCD displays, and we discussed a few of them earlier in the chapter. It would be ideal if one could simply look at a list of numbers and determine which display was best. Unfortunately, there is no industry-standard method for measuring these specifications. Without this standard, numbers are fairly useless. Furthermore, some manufacturers intentionally inflate theirs specs to attract those people who "buy numbers."

Fortunately, there are a couple of magazines that have done much of the work for you. *PC World* and *PC Magazine* both publish ratings of monitors that can help narrow the selection process by describing the strengths and weaknesses of each model on the list. Sometimes they also discuss the monitors that did not make the cut and why. Once the selection has been narrowed, it is time to use the best instruments for selecting a monitor — your eyes. Buying a monitor without looking at it critically is like buying a car without driving it. Even if the monitor is widely praised, it simply may not look good to you, and after all, you are going to be looking at it for a long time.

Once you have narrowed the selection to two or three models, it is time to go to your local computer store and see them in person. Most computer stores have a wall of monitors from which to choose. Be aware that it is unlikely that any of the monitors are set up correctly. Make sure that the store will allow you to put up images of your choosing and will allow you to optimize the monitor. The best way to do this is to use a program called DisplayMate. This excellent utility program is available directly from the publisher at www.displaymate.com, and it provides dozens of test patterns that are designed to establish the quality of a monitor. Different patterns are used for CRT and LCD displays and you will quickly become expert in discriminating among various products. DisplayMate also has a complementary set of patterns that are used to optimize the monitor at your work area once you have made a selection.

Now that you know how to choose a quality display, let's see how your eyes are affected by your choice. The next chapter will explore the visual aspect of viewing an electronic display and how it affects your eyes, specifically dealing with computer vision syndrome.

4

Computer Vision Syndrome

Jeffrey Anshel

CONTENTS

Introduction

Because computer use is such a high visually demanding task, vision problems and symptoms are very common. Most studies indicate that computer operators report more eye-related problems than noncomputer office workers. A number of investigators (Smith et al., 1981; Yamamoto, 1987; Dain et al., 1988; Collins et al., 1991) have indicated that visual symptoms occur in 75 to 90% of computer workers. In contrast, a survey released by the National Institute for Occupational Safety and Health (NIOSH) showed that only 22% of computer workers have musculoskeletal disorders.

A survey of optometrists (Sheedy, 1992) indicated that 10 million primary care eye examinations are given annually in this country, primarily because of visual problems at computers. This study eventually culminated in the compilation of the series of symptoms that are now collectively known as computer vision syndrome (CVS). This condition most often occurs when the viewing demand of the task exceeds the visual abilities of the computer user. The American Optometric Association defines CVS as that "complex of eye and vision problems related to near work that are experienced during or related to computer use." The symptoms can vary but mostly include eyestrain, headaches, blurred vision (distance or near), dry and irritated eyes, slow refocusing, neck and backache, light sensitivity, double vision, and color distortion.

The medical definition of a syndrome is the "aggregate signs and symptoms characteristic of a disease, a lesion, an anomaly, a type of a classification." While not technically being a true syndrome in the medical sense, CVS is a series of symptoms that are common to those who experience computer-related eye discomfort. Can someone who does not use a computer experience these symptoms? Yes they can! However, computer use has shown to increase the number and intensity of this series of symptoms presented to eyecare professionals. Thus, I believe that it should be addressed as an independent issue that must be resolved.

The causes for the inefficiencies and the visual symptoms are a combination of individual visual problems and poor office ergonomics. Poor office ergonomics can be further divided into poor workplace conditions and improper work habits. The above-mentioned survey also concluded that two thirds of the complaints were related to vision problems while one third were due to environmental factors. Many people have marginal vision disorders that do not cause symptoms when performing less demanding visual tasks. However, it has also been shown that computer users also have a higher incidence of complaints than noncomputer users in the same environment (Udo et al., 1991).

Let's review these symptoms and see if we can determine how they arise and how they may be addressed, both visually and environmentally.

Eyestrain

The eye care professions maintain a vague definition of eyestrain. One tends to think of a strain as what would happen to a muscle if it were overworked. In fact, it is rarely a strained muscle that causes the complaint of eyestrain.

The medical term for eyestrain is asthenopia (AS-then-OH-pee-ah), which itself is a rather vague term. The visual science dictionary defines asthenopia as the subjective complaint of uncomfortable, painful, and irritable vision. It then gives 24 different types of asthenopia based on various causes. Because of its subjectivity, however, it can have a myriad of meanings to any number of people. Asthenopia can be caused from some underlying conditions such as focusing spasm, different vision in each eye, astigmatism, hyperopia, myopia, excess light, voluntary focusing, eye coordination difficulties, and more.

When confronted with the complaint of eyestrain, it would be prudent to have a complete eye examination performed to determine the exact source of the complaint.

Headaches

Headaches are another of those asthenopic symptoms and are one of the primary reasons people seek an eye examination. They are also one of the most difficult maladies to diagnose and treat effectively. Headaches are reported at least once a month by 76% of women and 57% of men. There are numerous types of headaches and they can be caused by a number of different conditions. The International Headache Society classifies headaches in the following categories:

Migraine	Nonvascular intracranial disorder
Tension-type	Substance withdrawal
Cluster	Noncephalic infection
Miscellaneous unassociated with structural lesion	Metabolic disorder
Head trauma	Facial pain
Vascular disorders	Cranial neuralgia

It is beyond the scope of this book to delve into the various headache conditions and their origins. However, it would serve our purpose to distinguish between visual and nonvisual origin headaches and what might be the source of the symptom.

Visual headaches most often occur toward the front or sides of the head (there are a few exceptions to this); occur most often toward the middle or end of the day; do not appear upon awakening; do not produce visual auras of flashing lights; often occur in a different pattern (or not at all) on weekends than during the week; can occur on one side of the head more than the other; and bring other more general symptoms. It is, therefore, imperative to elicit a thorough case history to distinguish the type of headache involved. The worker should be queried about the time of onset, location of the pain, frequency, duration, severity, and precipitating factors such as stress, certain foods or medications. Associated signs and symptoms such as nausea, vomiting, light sensitivity, and noise sensitivity should also be noted.

Many times a worker will complain of a migraine headache. However, migraines are a very specific type of headache and have an organic, not visual, cause. There is no clinical diagnostic test to establish the presence of a migraine headache, so extensive laboratory tests would be appropriate. The worker should be referred for a neurological evaluation after all other variables have been accounted for.

Computer workers most likely get tension-type headaches. These can be precipitated by many forms of stress, including anxiety and depression; numerous eye conditions, including astigmatism and hyperopia; improper workplace conditions, including glare, poor lighting, and improper work-station setup. These types of headaches are mild to moderate in intensity, often occur on either or both sides of the head, are not aggravated by physical activity, develop during the early to middle part of the day, last from 30 minutes to the rest of the day, and are relieved by rest or sleep. Chronic tension headaches vary somewhat from this but have the same overall symptoms and occur much more frequently.

Visual and environmental conditions are the first places to look for a solution to a headache problem. If all obvious factors have been considered, medical management is in order, often starting with a complete eye examination to rule out a visual cause.

Blurred Vision

Visual acuity is the ability to distinguish between two distinctive points at a particular distance. This requires the image formed on the retina to be well circumscribed and distinct. If the image focuses in front of or behind the retina, it will strike the retina in an unfocused state, creating the subjective symptom of blur. This process is true for all distances with the viewing range of the human eye, which we routinely consider to be from within 20 feet to 16 inches.

We consider the 20-foot distance optical "infinity" due to the angulations of the light rays that emanate from that point. Whenever we direct our gaze to some point within 20 feet, we must activate our focusing mechanism to increase the focal power of the eye and regain the clear image on the retina. The ability of the eye to change its focal power is called accommodation and is dependent upon age. Therefore, we must consider many factors when discussing the accommodative ability of the individual.

Blurred vision symptoms can result from refractive error (e.g., hyperopia, myopia, astigmatism), improper prescription lenses, presbyopia, or other focusing disorders. Wiggins and Daum (1991) found that small amounts of refractive error contribute to the visual discomfort of computer users. Considering the working environment, blurred images can also arise from a dirty screen, poor viewing angle, reflected glare, or a poor quality or defective monitor. All of these factors should be considered when this symptom occurs.

While viewing an object at a near (or intermediate) viewing distance of less than 20 feet, the eyes must accommodate. The point of focus is often times not directly at the point of the object but usually behind it at some short distance. As the computer worker views the task for an extended

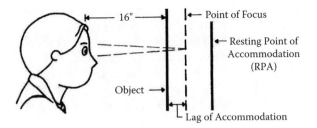

FIGURE 4.1
The "lag of accommodation" is the point to which the eye actually focuses, usually behind the target being viewed.

period of time, this lag of accommodation increases, often leading to a subjective symptom of blur. The eyes must then expend more effort to pull the focusing point back to the screen. If this is accomplished with enough effort, then the symptom might become a headache; if not accomplished well enough, blurred vision might be the symptom.

A condition known as transient myopia has been shown to be more prevalent in a population of computer users. This is a condition in which a person exhibits myopia toward the end of the day but not at any other times. Many times, the myopia is not present early in the day or on weekends. One study (Luberto et al., 1989) found that 20% of computer workers had a nearsighted tendency toward the end of their work shift. Watten and Lie (1992) confirmed this study when they found 30 computer workers who had this myopic trend after two to four hours of work. However, another study of transient myopia (Rosenfeld and Ciuffreda, 1994) showed that this condition also occurs after normal near-point viewing of a printed target. Studies showing permanent myopic changes have not shown this to be a concern at this time. However, many of those studies suffer from a lack of adequate control groups and low numbers of population tested.

Glare is also a concern because of the eye attending to the glare image rather than the screen image. If a specular reflection is noticeable on the screen, the eye will attempt to focus on it. The image of the glare source will appear to be somewhere behind the screen (much as your image is reflected in a mirror) and the screen image can appear blurred. This can become more noticeable as computer usage time is increased.

Dry and Irritated Eyes

The front surface of the eye is covered with a tissue that consists of many glands. These glands secrete the tears that cover the eye surface and keep the eye moist, which is necessary for normal eye function. The tears help maintain the proper oxygen balance of the external eye structures and to keep the optical properties of the eye sharp. The normal tear layer is cleaned off and refreshed by the blinking action of the eyelids.

The blink reflex is one of the fastest reflexes in the body and is present at birth. However, our blink rate varies with different activities — faster when we are very active, slower when we are sedate or concentrating. Yaginuma et al. (1990) measured the blink rate and tearing on four computer workers and noted that the blink rate dropped very significantly during work at a computer compared with before and after work. There was no significant change in tearing. Patel et al. (1991) measured blink rate by directly observing a group of 16 subjects. The mean blink rate during conversation was 18.4 blinks per minute, and during computer use it dropped to 3.6 — more than a five-fold decrease! Tsubota and Nakamori (1993) measured blink rates on 104 office workers. The mean blink rates were 22 blinks per minute under relaxed conditions, 10 blinks while reading a book on a table, and only 7 while viewing text on a computer. Their data support the fact that blink rate decreases during computer use, but also show that other tasks can decrease the blink rate.

Possible explanations for the decreased blink rate include concentration on the task or a relatively limited range of eye movements. Although both book reading and computer work result in significantly decreased blink rates, a difference between them is that computer work usually requires a higher gaze angle, resulting in an increased rate of tear evaporation. Tsubota and Nakamori (1993) measured a mean exposed eye surface of 2.2 cm^2, while subjects were relaxed, 1.2 cm^2 while reading a book on the table, and 2.3 cm^2 while working at a computer. The size of the eye opening is related to the direction of gaze, as we gaze higher, the eyes open wider. Since the primary route of tear elimination is through evaporation and the amount of evaporation roughly relates to eye opening, the higher gaze angle when viewing a computer screen results in faster tear loss. It is also likely that the higher gaze angle results in a greater percentage of blinks that are incomplete. It has been suggested that incomplete blinks are not effective because the tear layer being replenished is defective and not a full tear layer. The exposed ocular surface area has been shown to be one of the most important indices of visual ergonomics (Sotoyama et al., 1995).

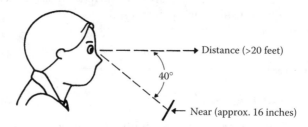

FIGURE 4.2
The variation of eye blink rate on various viewing tasks. (Tsubota and Nakamore, 1993)

An additional factor that can contribute to dry eye is that office air environment is often low in humidity and can contain contaminants. This has been noted as a possible cause of Sick Building Syndrome. Additionally, the static electricity generated by the display screen itself attracts dust particles into the immediate area. These can also contribute to particulate matter entering the eyes, leading to dry eye symptoms.

Neck and Back Ache

This book is about the visual aspects of computer use — so why a section on neck and back problems? It is often said in medical circles that "the eyes lead the body." Nature has made our visual system so dominant that we will alter our body posture to accommodate any deficiency in the way we see. One example often referred to is that of the young piano student who is giving his/her first recital — a very stressful situation. If a wrong note is played, the first reaction is to squint the eyes and lean in toward the music to confirm what the note should have been. This is a classic example of how the auditory feedback (the wrong sound) triggers a visual response (the squint) that leads to a postural change (the lean). Galinsky et al. (1993) found that subjects monitoring a visual display reported greater subjective fatigue than those monitoring an auditory display.

A similar situation can be seen in many office situations where the vision of a worker is compromised and they must adapt their posture to ease the strain on the visual system. If an older worker is using reading glasses (single vision), which are designed for a 16-inch viewing distance, they must lean in toward a screen that may be 20 to 25 inches away in order to clear the image. If the same worker is using traditional bifocals, which are designed to see the near object in the lower visual field, they must tilt their head backward and lean forward to put the viewing section of the lens into proper position to see the screen. If a computer worker is most often viewing hard copy that is off to one side, they might need to keep moving their head back and forth to view the screen alternatively with the hard copy. This will also lead to neck discomfort. This same condition can exist if the computer user is not a touch-typist. They will continually alternate their viewing gaze between the keyboard and the screen using head movements, which can cause neck and shoulder fatigue.

These and many other situations are all too common in the office environment and cause excessive postural accommodations that lead to the symptoms of neck and back discomfort. Lie and Watten (1994) found that doing computer work for three hours contributed not only to eye muscle fatigue but also muscle pain in the head, neck and upper back regions. Fahrback and Chapman (1990) found the highest area of complaints for heavy computer users was the head and for light computer users was the back. One

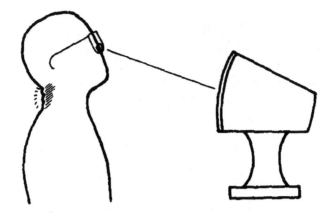

FIGURE 4.3
Bifocal lenses require the wearer to gaze downward in order to properly see through the reading portion of the lens. This will necessitate a head tilt if the gaze angle is too high.

of the main reasons for these problems is the setup of the workstation — most often the position of the monitor. All too frequently the monitor is placed either on top of the Central Processing Unit (CPU) or on a monitor stand. This places the screen in a position where the user must look either straight ahead or actually upward in their gaze.

Ankrum et al. (1994) have done extensive work in this area of viewing angle and eye position. They discuss how eye level is often determined with the user sitting "tall." However, in normal, upright sitting (without a visual target), Hsiao and Keyserling (1991) found that subjects tilted their head and neck an average of 13 degrees forward from the upright position. If the monitor is set to eye level, the user is presented with a choice: either assume a more erect head and neck posture than preferred or employ a gaze angle above the reference line which passes through the right ear hole and the lowest part of the right eye socket (Frankfurt line).

When the head-erect posture becomes tiring, users have limited possibilities for relief. One option is to tilt the head backward (extension). Hill and Kroemer (1986) found that when users in an upright-seated posture were shown targets 50 to 100 cm away, they preferred to gaze an average of 29 degrees below the Frankfurt line. Another alternative posture available to computer users with eye-level monitors is the forward head position, in which the head remains erect while jutting forward from the trunk. Users sometimes assume a forward head posture in a counterproductive attempt to relieve muscle tension caused by contracted neck muscles (Mackinnon and Novak, 1994).

The last alternative neck posture available with an erect trunk position is flexion, or forward bending. Chaffin (1973) found that 15 degrees of sustained neck flexion for a long period (six hours with 10 minute breaks each hour) resulted in no elevated electro-muscular reading or subjective reports

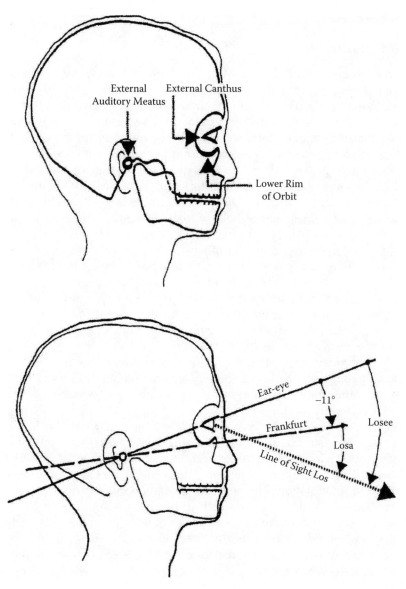

External Auditory Meatus

External Canthus

Lower Rim of Orbit

Ear-eye

−11°

Frankfurt

Losee

Losa

Line of Sight Los

FIGURE 4.4
The Frankfurt line.

of discomfort. Sustained neck tilts of more than 30 degrees, however, greatly increased neck fatigue rates.

There are many schools of thought as to the perfect height for the screen and each has its own supporting theories. These will be discussed in further detail in Chapter 6.

Light Sensitivity

The eyes are designed to be stimulated by light and to control the amount of light entering the eyeball. There are, however, conditions that exist today that are foreign to the natural lighting environment and can cause an adverse reaction to light. The largest single factor in the workplace is glare. Glare will be discussed in more detail in regard to the remedies for the workplace but it bears some discussion here because it is a significant factor in CVS.

There are two general categories of glare: discomfort glare and reflective glare. This section will discuss discomfort glare because it is the more common cause for light sensitivity. Discomfort glare is largely caused by large disparities in brightness in the field of view. It is much more desirable to eliminate bright sources of light from the field of view and strive to obtain a relatively even distribution of luminances. A person is at greater risk to experience discomfort glare when the source has a higher luminance and when it is closer to the point of attention.

One of the primary reasons discomfort glare is a problem for computer users is that light often leaves the overhead fluorescent fixture in a wide angle, resulting in light directly entering the worker's eyes. It is very common for the luminance of the fixture to be more than 100 times greater than that of the display screen that the worker is viewing. This is a particular problem of computer workers because they are looking horizontally in the room (assuming the screen is at eye level). Bright open windows pose the same risks as overhead light fixtures.

Workers are also at risk for discomfort glare if they use a dark background display screen, resulting in a greater luminance disparity between the task and other objects in the room. Alternately, if a newer LCD panel is used, the brightness of the background on the screen might be too intense for the surrounding illumination. The newer LCD displays offer brightness in the range of 250 to 300 cd/m^2 or more, which is much brighter than a common CRT luminance of 120 cd/m^2. Other sources of large luminance disparity at the computer workstation include white paper on the desk, light-colored desk surfaces, and desk lamps directed toward the eyes or which illuminate the desk area too highly.

More details on lighting are discussed in Chapter 5.

Double Vision

In Chapter 2 we discussed the process of binocular vision and how we manage to see just one image while using two eyes. This normal viewing process can be disturbed by excess use, especially when looking at a close working distance for extended periods of time. When we lose our ability to maintain the "lock" between the eyes, they can misalign and aim at different points in space. If both eyes keep transmitting the image back to the brain, we will experience double vision, or diplopia (di-PLO-pee-ah).

Double vision is a very uncomfortable and unacceptable condition for our visual system. We will most likely suppress or turn off the image of one eye rather than experience the double images. When viewing a near-point object, the extraocular muscles converge the line of sight of the eyes inward toward the nose. Convergence allows the eyes to maintain the alignment of the image on corresponding retinal cells in each eye.

We previously discussed the resting point of accommodation (Chapter 2) but there is also a resting point of convergence. This point varies among individuals but the average is about 100 cm (Jaschinski-Kruza, 1991). Looking at objects closer than one's resting point causes strain on the muscles controlling the vergence. The closer the distance, the greater the strain (Collins, 1975). In fact, the resting point of convergence has an even greater impact on eyestrain than the resting point of accommodation. Jaschinski-Kruza (1988) measured productivity on a group of subjects, which was at its maximum at the 100 cm distance. Owens and Wolf-Kelly (1987) found that after one hour of near work, the resting points of both accommodation and vergence demonstrated an inward shift. The magnitude of the shifts depended on the positions before the near work — subjects with initial far resting points exhibited the greatest inward shifts.

While these studies seem to point to the significance of the resting point of convergence, it has yet to become a standard office testing procedure. Until it does, eye care professionals will continue to perform standard binocular vision tests to determine near-point visual abilities.

Oftentimes a worker will not experience this doubling of vision while using the computer but afterward. This is a sign that the convergence system is working, but is unable to stop working! If the resting point of vergence is so far inward that distance objects cannot be viewed properly, they might appear to double. Fortunately, this problem is not predominant, mainly due to the visual system's "survival" instinct and suppression ability. However, it is unfortunate as well because the symptom of this type of stress may not be noticeable until it reaches an advanced stage. This is further evidence for the need for periodic eye examinations that can determine workers' vergence abilities.

After-Images and Color Distortion

Anyone who had his or her picture taken with a camera with flash attachment has seen an after-image. It is that persistent image of the light that we still see for some time after the initial flash has gone. It is beyond the scope of this book to discuss the physiological reasons for this effect but it is normally of no consequence because it dissipates within a short time. It has, however, been reported in some cases of computer users who have looked at an excessively bright screen for an extended period of time.

Our retina is also responsible for our perception of color vision. Although we still have only a theory of color vision, we have a pretty good idea of how it works. There are three types of cones in the retina that mediate colors (red, blue, and green), and when they are exposed to a particular color for an extended period of time, they become bleached, or desensitized, to that color. Since those cones are temporarily nonfunctional, the other neighboring cones become more effective and they produce a color that is complementary to the original bleaching color. This condition is called the McCullough effect (McCullough, 1965). For example, looking at the color green for a long time will exhibit a red (or pinkish) after-image when looking at a white surface. This has been demonstrated in almost 20% of computer users in a study (Seaber et al., 1987), but there was no permanent damage, and it could not be determined who is more likely to experience the effect. Working on a full-color monitor with various colors used throughout a day will likely not create this condition.

Computer vision syndrome is a technological by-product of excessive viewing of computer screens without regard to common sense visual hygiene. By just using some common sense and education about the visual system, the symptoms of CVS can be diminished or eliminated.

References

Ankrum, D.R. and Nemeth, K.J. Constrained neck postures with eye-level computers, Private correspondence, 1994.

Chaffin, D.B. Localized muscle fatigue — definition and measurement, *Journal of Occupational Medicine*, 15, (4) 346–354, 1973.

Collins, C.C. et al. Muscle strain during unrestrained human eye movements, *Journal of Physiology*, 245, 351–369, 1975.

Collins, M.J. et al. Task variables and visual discomfort associated with the use of computers, *Optometry and Visual Science*, 68:1, 27–33, 1991.

Dain S.J. et al. Symptoms in VDU operators, *American Journal of Optometry and Physiological Optics*, 6, 162–167, 1988.

Fahrback, P.A. and Chapman, L.J. Computer work duration and musculoskeletal discomfort, *AAOHN Journal*, 38 (1), 32–36, 1990.

Galinsky, T.L. et al. Psychophysical determinants of stress in sustained attention, *Human Factors*, 35 (4), 603–614, 1993.

Hill, S.G. and Kroemer, K.H.E. Preferred declination of the line of sight, *Human Factors*, 28, (2), 127–134, 1986.

Hsiao, H. and Keyserling, W.M. Evaluating posture behavior during seated tasks, *International Journal of Industrial Ergonomics*, 8, 313–334, 1991.

Jaschinski-Krusza, W. Visual strain during VDU work: The effect of viewing distance and dark focus, *Ergonomics*, 31 (10), 1449–1465, 1988.

Jaschinski-Krusza, W. Eyestrain in VDU users: Viewing distance and the resting position of ocular muscles, *Human Factors*, 33, (1), 69–83, 1991.

Lie, I. and Watten, R.G. Computer work, oculomotor strain and subjective complaints: An experimental and clinical study, *Ergonomics*, 37 (8), 1419–1433, 1994.

Luberto, F. et al. Temporary myopia and subjective symptoms in video display terminal operators, *Med Lav*, 80(2): 155–163, 1989.

Mackinnon, S.E. and Novak, C.B. Clinical commentary: Pathogenesis of cumulative trauma disorder, *Journal of Hand Surgery*, 19A, (5), 873–883, 1994.

McCullough, C. Color adaptation of edge detectors in the human visual system, *Science*, 149, 1115, 1965.

Owens, D.A. and Wolf-Kelly, K. Near work, visual fatigue and variations of oculomotor tonus. *Investigative Ophthalmology and Visual Science*, 28, 743–749, 1987.

Patel, S. et al. Effect of visual display unit use on blink rate and tear stability, *Optometry and Visual Science*, 68(11), 888–892, 1991.

Rosenfeld, M. and Ciuffreda, KJ. Cognitive demand and transient near-work-induced myopia, *Optometry and Visual Science*, 71(6); 475–481, 1994.

Seaber, J.H. et al. Incidence and characteristics of McCullough aftereffects following video display terminal use, *Journal of Occupational Medicine*, 29: 9, 727–729; 1987.

Sheedy, J.E. Vision problems at video display terminals: A survey of optometrists, *Journal of American Optometric Association*, 63, 687–692, 1992.

Smith, M.J. et al. An Investigation of health complaints and job stress in video display operations, *Human Factors*, 23 (4), 387–400, 1981.

Sotoyama, M. et al. Ocular surface area as an informative index of visual ergonomics, *Industrial Health*, 33:2, 43–55, 1995.

Tsubota, K. and Nakamori, K. Dry eyes and video display terminals, *New England Journal of Medicine*, 328, 8, 1993.

Udo, H. et al. Visual load of working with visual display terminal — introduction of COMPUTER to newspaper editing and visual effect, *Journal of Human Ergonomics*, 20:2, 109–121, 1991.

Watten, R.G. and Lie, I. Time factors in computer-induced myopia and visual fatigue: an experimental study, *Journal of Human Ergonomics*, 21(1): 13–20, 1992.

Wiggins, N.P. and Daum K.M. Visual discomfort and astigmatic refractive errors in use, *Journal of American Optometric Association*, 62 (9), 680–684, 1991.

Yagunuma, Y. et al. Study of the relationship between lacrimation and blink in work, *Ergonomics*, 33(6), 799–809, 1990.

Yamamoto, S. Visual, musculoskeletal and neuropsychological health complaints of workers using video display terminal and an occupational health guideline, *Japan Journal of Ophthalmology*, 31:1, 171–183, 1987.

5

Office Lighting for Computer Use

James E. Sheedy

CONTENTS

Introduction

This chapter discusses some of the fundamental aspects of light, its effects upon the eye, the measurement of light, and office lighting principles. It should go without saying that good lighting is important for visual efficiency and comfort. Improper lighting is probably the biggest environmental factor that contributes to visual discomfort. The topic of lighting can become complex, and good lighting is difficult to define. However, there are a couple of important conclusions about office lighting that can be stated at the beginning:

- Although it is necessary and important to have an adequate amount of light, most computer workplaces have enough light. In fact, as discussed later, there is often too much light in the office environment. Inadequate illumination levels are usually not a problem for computer users.

- Light distribution is more commonly a problem for computer users. The most common lighting problem for computer users is glare from bright lights or objects in the field of view.

Lights

The Eye and Light

Of course, without light, there is no vision. However, even more fundamentally, we can say that without the eye there is no light. Light is actually defined based upon the sensitivity of the eye and visual system to electromagnetic radiation. Without the eye and visual system, there is only electromagnetic radiation.

The relative sensitivity of the eye is shown graphically in Figure 5.1. It may be seen that the peak sensitivity of the eye is at 555 nanometers (nm), or 10^{-9} meters. At wavelengths 510 nm and 610 nm, the relative sensitivity of the eye is only about 50% of the sensitivity at 555 nm. This means that

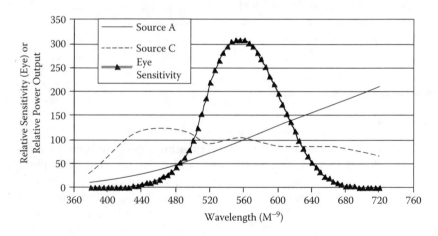

FIGURE 5.1
The relative sensitivity of the eye, and the relative outputs of Source A (tungsten light) and Source C (sunlight).

twice as much energy is required at 510 nm (or 610 nm) compared with 555 nm in order to have the same magnitude of light — or to create the same level of perceived brightness. At wavelengths 430 nm and 685 nm, the eye sensitivity is only about 1% of the sensitivity at the peak of 555 nm.

Lamp Types and Characteristics

Figure 5.1 also shows the distributions of standard source A (similar to the standard tungsten lights in our lamps at home) and of standard source C (similar to sunlight). The tungsten source has a considerably larger proportion of its output in the red end of the spectrum, whereas the light from the sun has a more equal output across the visible spectrum. Both of these are continuous spectra — i.e., they both produce radiation at all of the wavelengths to which the eye is sensitive. This is an important feature for good color rendition of objects. This is because objects in the environment just reflect the light impinging upon them, and the percentage of light reflected by the object depends upon the wavelength of the light. Light sources with continuous spectra, such as A and C in Figure 5.1, effectively "sample" the entire spectral reflectance characteristics of objects. As result, these continuous spectra enable small differences in the reflectance characteristics of objects to be identified — i.e., they result in better color discrimination and color rendering of objects.

The efficiency of light sources largely depends upon the extent to which electrical energy (watts) is converted to light energy (lumens). The ideal light source, from an efficiency point of view, would be one in which all of the electrical energy was converted to output at 555nm. The light source that comes closest to this situation is a low-pressure sodium lamp in which all of the output is at 589 nm. This lamp type has an approximate efficiency of 200 lumens/watt. Low-pressure sodium lamps produce a very saturated yellow color and are often used for outdoor lighting around buildings. Unfortunately, the monochromatic nature of the low-pressure sodium means that the light reflected from each object also contains only 1 wavelength, and the reflected light from each object is determined only by its reflectance at 589 nm. Because the only light reflected from all objects is 589 nm, objects cannot be distinguished on the basis of their wavelength spectrum — i.e., there is effectively no color vision with this light source. Discontinuous spectra, the extreme example of which is low-pressure sodium, provide poorer color discrimination and color rendition; than continuous sources. Low-pressure sodium light sources are almost never used indoors because of the extremely poor color rendition, they are typically only used in outdoor situations where color discrimination is not required and where the high efficiency is important. High-pressure sodium lamps have a broader spectral output than low-pressure sodium, although it still does not contain all spectral wavelengths. High-pressure sodium lamps provide high efficiency (100 to 140 lumens/watt) and also allow some color rendering (however, less than typical indoor lighting), and hence are used widely for outdoor lighting.

Tungsten lamps (i.e., source A in Figure 5.1) are not very efficient (8 to 20 lumens/watt) primarily because of the high-energy output in the red and infrared end of the spectrum. The infrared output, which is not visible, converts to heat instead of light — the heat of tungsten lamps is wasted energy. The low efficiency and large heat output, which must be compensated with air conditioning in summer months, are reasons that tungsten lighting is seldom used in offices. Tungsten lamps provide very good color rendition because of their continuous spectrum and provide pleasant lighting that is considered "warm" because of the high red content, so they are very good choices for personal living spaces.

Lighting

Fluorescent lamps are used most frequently in offices because they provide a good combination of efficiency and color rendering properties. All fluorescent lamps have mercury vapor within the tube that emits radiation at only wavelengths 406, 436, 546, and 579 nm. The output spectra of fluorescent lamps (shown in Figure 5.2) each have large outputs at these wavelengths. The inner side of the glass tube is coated with a phosphor that absorbs energy emitted by the mercury vapor and then re-emits it, always at a longer wavelength according to the laws of physics. The continuous output in between the mercury lines shown in Figure 5.2 is from the phosphor. Different phosphors are used to create different spectral outputs. Fluorescent tubes are considerably more efficient than tungsten because less output is wasted on nonvisible regions. The color rendering properties of fluorescent lamps are also quite good, although because of the output spikes of the underlying mercury vapor it is not as good as tungsten.

A summary of typical lamp characteristics is provided in Table 5.1. The color temperature (CT) can be characterized as representing the red/blue balance of the light output; lower numbers have more red output and are "warmer" psychologically. Natural light from outdoors ranges from about 5500 to 8000 degrees Kelvin (K), and tungsten lamps range from 2600 to 3000 K; lower wattage bulbs usually have lower color temperatures. The CTs of fluorescent lamps generally fall between natural light and tungsten. Color temperature can affect the mood of the environment. A CT of 3000 K is considered warm and typical of friendly and intimate environments such as better restaurants, libraries, boutiques, etc.; 3500 K could be considered neutral and good for many offices, reception areas, and shops; 4000 K is considered cool and is also used in many office environments, mass merchandising stores, classrooms, etc.; 4500 K and higher color temperatures are considered brighter and are used in many public places. The color-rendering index is calculated on the basis of how well the source reproduces eight standard

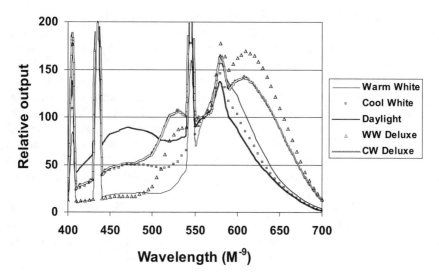

FIGURE 5.2
Relative spectral output of common fluorescent lamps.

TABLE 5.1

Typical Properties of Lamp Types

Lamp Type	Efficiency (lumens/watt)	Color Temperature (°K)	Color Rendering Index
Tungsten	10–40	2600-3000	100
Low pressure sodium	200	n/a	0
High pressure sodium	100–140	2100	25
Fluorescent			
Warm white	80	3000	70
Warm white deluxe	50–80	3000	85
Cool white	80	4100	70
Cool white deluxe	50–60	4100	85
Daylight	50–60	6500	85

color chips. The primary advantage of the deluxe fluorescent lamps is increased color rendering compared to nondeluxe.

High-Frequency Ballasts — Fluorescent Lamps

To produce light in a fluorescent bulb, an arc of electricity passes through the mercury vapor causing it to emit radiation. The function of the ballast is to produce a high voltage to begin the electrical current through the tube, and then to reduce the voltage because lesser voltage is required to keep the current flowing and continued high voltage would burn out the tube.

Because line voltage is 60 Hertz AC (50 Hz in Europe) the arc of electricity moves one way and then the other through the tube 60 times per second. This produces 60 Hz flicker at the ends of the tube and 120 Hz flicker in the middle of the tube. The threshold for human detection of flicker is generally 30 to 50 Hz; hence the flicker from normally ballasted fluorescent tubes cannot usually be perceived. However, there is considerable evidence that flicker rates higher than those that are perceived are received physiologically (Berman et al., 1991; Eyesel, 1984; Murata et al., 1991) and are also associated with symptoms of discomfort (Wilkins et al., 1989). There is also evidence that flicker rates above the perception threshold affect eye movements (Wilkins, 1986) and also cause short-term changes in some visual functions (Laubli et al., 1986; Harwood and Foley, 1987).

High frequency electronic ballasts convert the 60 Hz frequency to 20 to 50 KHz. The considerably higher flicker rate removes the possibility that it is detrimental to vision or comfort. The high-frequency ballast also improves lamp efficiency and reduces audible hum from the ballast.

Light Units and Measurements

Illumination

Illumination is the amount of light (lumens) falling on a surface (area). The common units of illumination are foot-candles (lumens/square foot of surface) and lux (lumens/square meter of surface). One square meter contains 10.76 square feet, therefore 10.76 lux is the same amount of illumination as 1 fc, i.e., this conversion gives the same light density per area. A common and convenient conversion is 10 lux = 1 fc. The lighting in a room is typically designed to provide a predetermined illumination level. A meter that measures illumination is often simply called a "light meter." The light meter contains a sensor that is placed at the location at which a measure of illumination is desired. Sometimes the sensing device is an integral part of the unit and sometimes it extends from it with a wire attachment. The measure of illumination can vary quite significantly at different locations within the same room. It will depend upon height within the room, location with respect to light fixtures, and shadows (make sure your own shadow does not affect the measurement). For office work, the illumination at desk level is usually most pertinent. Illumination is usually measured on horizontal surfaces; therefore the measuring device should be oriented horizontally. For measuring illumination on the surface of a computer display the measuring device should be oriented parallel to the display surface.

Higher illumination levels are required for more demanding visual tasks. This is because human visual discrimination abilities continue to improve with more light (Sheedy et al., 1984). Suggested illumination levels (ANSI,

TABLE 5.2

Suggested Illumination Levels Based upon Visual Task Demands

Illumination Level (fc)	Task Description
2–5	Public spaces with dark surroundings
5–10	Simple orientation tasks or short visits
10–20	Working spaces with infrequent tasks
20–50	Tasks with high contrast or large size
50–100	Tasks with medium contrast or small size
100–200	Tasks with low contrast and very small size
200–500	Low contrast and very small size — prolonged viewing
500–1000	Very prolonged and exacting tasks
1000–2000	Extremely critical and exacting tasks

1993) are provided in Table 5.2. It is also well known that with age greater lighting levels are required. Those aged 55 and older can require twice as much light as a 20-year-old for the same tasks.

Luminance

Luminance, the other important measure of light, is a measure of the amount of light coming toward the eye from an object (per angular area of the object). The common unit of luminance is candle/square meter (cd/m^2). The eye responds directly to the luminance of objects — we judge the brightness of objects based upon their luminance. On the other hand, the eye does not directly sense illumination. Illumination is important to the eye insofar as greater illumination results in greater amounts of light reflecting from objects; hence the luminance of the objects (i.e., light reflected into the eye by the object) is increased.

The relationship between luminance and brightness is not linear but logarithmic. Each subsequent "step" in perceptual brightness requires a greater amount of additional luminance than did the previous step. This is similar to most other human sensory scaling such as sound and touch. The result of this nonlinear scaling is that our visual system is good at determining whether one object is brighter or dimmer than another (1%), but not good at judging the magnitude of luminance. A practical example is that the luminance of a computer display may be 100 cd/m^2 and a sunny sidewalk seen through a window may be 6000 cd/m^2, but the sidewalk does not subjectively appear even close to 60 times brighter than the computer display.

Luminance is measured with a luminance meter or photometer. Using a photometer is similar to sighting through a camera; in fact, the built-in light meter within a camera is actually a crude luminance meter. The user sees a circular reticule or "measuring circle." The meter should be aimed so that this measuring circle is located on the object for which the luminance measurement is desired. For a valid measurement, the entire measuring circle should be filled with the object being measured. The luminance of an object

TABLE 5.3

Typical Luminance Levels in a Computer Workstation
Environment*

Visual Object	Luminance (cd/m²)
Dark background computer display	20–25
Light background computer display	80–120
White reference page with 75 fc illumination	200
White reference page with desk lamp	400
Window — blue sky	2500
Window — concrete in sun	6000–12000
Fluorescent lamps — poor design	1000–5000
Desk lamp — direct viewing	1500–10000

   * Note, however, that actual measurement in any given workstation en-
     vironment may differ greatly from those listed.

will depend upon the angle from which it is viewed if it has a specular or
glass-like component to its reflection characteristics. For example, the luminance (or brightness) of metal or glossy paper sitting on a table can change
quite significantly if viewed from a different angle. Therefore, in computer-
using environments, it is usually best to make measurements from the normal location of the computer user's eyes. Typical luminance ranges in a
computer workstation are shown in Table 5.3.

Glare Discomfort

Definition and Quantification

High luminance levels in the field of view create glare discomfort. This is a
well-known phenomenon. The threshold sizes and locations of visual stimuli
that cause glare discomfort have been determined (Guth, 1981), however the
physiological basis for glare discomfort is not known. Because large luminance disparities in the field of view can cause glare discomfort, it is best to
have a visual environment in which the luminances of objects within the
field of view are relatively equal.

Because of glare discomfort, the Illuminating Engineering Society (IES,
1989) has established, and ANSI has accepted (ANSI/IESNA RP-1-1993)
certain maximum luminance ratios that should not be exceeded. The luminance ratio between the central task and the immediate visual surroundings
(within a radius of 25 degrees) should not exceed 1:3 or 3:1. The luminance
ratio between the task and more remote visual surroundings (beyond 25
degrees) should not exceed 1:10 or 10:1. Glare sources are more bothersome
when they have higher luminance and when they are closer to the fixation
point.

Because of glare discomfort, the distribution of luminance in the field of view of the computer user is the most important aspect of lighting insofar as the visual system is concerned. The geometry of the lighting is akin to the quality of the lighting. This light geometry is affected by the lamp type, luminaire (light unit or fixture) design, how the light is further directed into the office through the use of baffles, blinds, drapes, etc., and how it is reflected from the various surfaces in the room such as walls, ceilings, and furniture. Good lighting is accomplished when all of the visual objects in the field of view have nearly equal brightness, i.e., they all are similar in luminance. Bad lighting occurs when objects in the field of view have great differences in luminance.

General lighting principle for visual comfort: eliminate bright lights from the field of view and strive to obtain a relatively even distribution of luminance (brightness) in the field of view.

With a luminance meter or photometer it is easy to determine whether the luminance ratios within a given work environment fall within the ANSI guidelines by measuring the luminance levels of objects from the eye location of the worker. There are many objects in the field of view that can cause luminance ratios in excess of those recommended by the ANSI/IES. For a computer user, the luminance of the screen should be measured first because this is the primary task and usually sets the lower end of the luminance ratio. It may be seen from the typical values in Table 5.3 that windows and overhead lights can easily exceed the 3:1 and 10:1 ratios.

Because the luminance level of white background displays is closer to those of other objects in the work environment, white background displays will typically result in lower luminance ratios than dark background displays and hence are more comfortable. In the earlier days of computing when dark background displays were commonplace, it was often recommended that light levels in offices with computers be lower than usual. This was because the display brightness could not really be increased, so the next best solution was to reduce the overall brightness of the office in order to reduce luminance ratios. White background displays are a better fit for the general luminance levels in typical offices. The best way to adjust the brightness of a computer display is to adjust it to generally match the immediate visual surroundings of the display.

Another problem that occurs with large disparities in the brightness of objects in the field of view is transient adaptation. When looking from brighter objects to darker objects or vice versa, there is a brief period of time after the eye movement during which the eye has to adapt to the new brightness level. This is most apparent when entering or leaving a dark movie theater or restaurant in the daytime. These are situations in which the eye needs to completely adapt to a different range of brightness. This same effect occurs on a smaller scale when the eye needs to fixate back and forth from bright to dark objects in a given environment. This can be especially bothersome if the luminance levels of reference document and computer display are disparate.

Luminaires and Glare

Windows and overhead lights are a particular problem for computer workers who are generally gazing horizontally in the room. Other common sources of glare at the computer workstation include white paper on the desk, white desktop surfaces, and desk lamps aimed towards the eye or that illuminate the desk area too greatly.

Possibly the most common source of discomfort glare is shown in the Figure 5.3. Many luminaires distribute light widely, i.e., there is a broad range of angles from which the light leaves the fixture. This has the advantage that the spacing between fixtures can be relatively large in order to provide even distribution of light throughout the room, i.e., fewer fixtures are required. However, the wide angle of distribution results in light directly entering the eyes of computer workers. It is very common for the luminance of the fixture to be more than 100 times that of the computer display the worker is viewing — far exceeding the ANSI IES recommended maximum luminance ratio of 10:1.

Good lighting design can significantly reduce discomfort glare. The luminaire can be designed so that light leaves the fixture in a narrower range of angles, thereby not directly entering the eyes of the computer user (Figure 5.4). This is most commonly accomplished with parabolic shaped louvers in the luminaire. The disadvantage of this approach is that the luminaires must be more closely spaced in order to provide even illumination across the room, thereby requiring more fixtures per room. An even better solution is indirect lighting (Figure 5.5) in which the light is bounced off the ceiling, resulting in a large low luminance source of light for the room. Indirect lighting

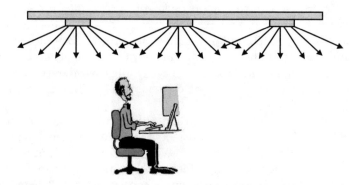

FIGURE 5.3
Luminaires with wide angle of light distribution. Light from fixture directly enters eyes of computer user, hence the fixture appears very bright and causes glare discomfort.

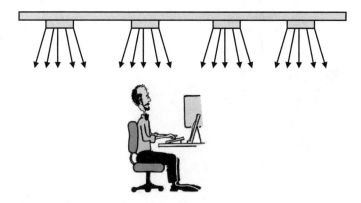

FIGURE 5.4
Luminaires with parabolic louvers and resulting narrow angle of light distribution. Light does not directly enter the eyes of the computer user.

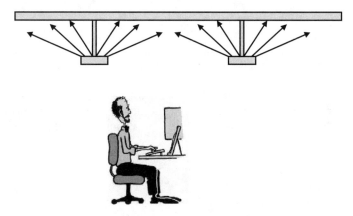

FIGURE 5.5
Indirect lighting in which light is reflected from the ceiling — light does not directly enter the eyes of the computer user.

eliminates overhead glare and also allows wider spacing of the fixtures. However, indirect lighting requires that the fixtures be hung 12 to 18 in. below the ceiling, thereby requiring slightly greater ceiling height.

Testing for Glare Discomfort

The easiest way to test for glare discomfort is with the visor test shown in Figure 5.6. View the computer display from the normal eye location and be aware of any bright lights in the peripheral visual field. Use the hand or something like a file folder to shield the eyes and note whether there is an immediate sense of improved visual comfort. If the test is positive, then the lights that were blocked are a source of glare discomfort. Most people, when

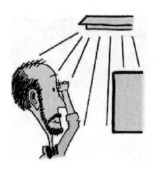

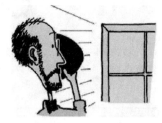

FIGURE 5.6

The visor test. Temporarily block light from the eyes with the hand or other baffle, an immediate sensation of comfort by eliminating the light indicates that glare discomfort is present.

performing this test in the presence of bright overhead fluorescent lights, will notice the glare discomfort. If an immediate improvement in comfort is appreciated, then the cumulative effects of an entire workday are understandable.

Measurement Method

A luminance meter can be used to test for glare discomfort by measuring the luminance of key objects in the field of view to determine if they exceed the ANSI/IES ratios of 3:1 and 10:1. Measurements should be made with the photometer viewing from approximately the same location as the user's eyes. It is best to use a fairly large aperture size (about 1 degree) so that the spatially averaged luminance value of a given stimulus can be determined. The luminance levels of detail (e.g., the luminance of the individual text letters) are not as important as the mean luminance of larger areas within the visual field. Measure the luminance level of the screen, the reference document, wall or desk area behind computer, general office luminance, desk lamp, window, and overhead lights. For each measurement note the angle between the normal line of sight to the computer and the line toward the glare source. This angle can be measured or estimated by viewing the computer user from the side and viewing the geometry through a clear protractor. The luminance ratios of the peripheral objects to the computer display can then be calculated and compared with the maximum recommended luminance ratios of 1:3 or 3:1 between the task and the immediate visual surroundings (within 25 degrees) and 1:10 or 10:1 between the task and more remote visual surroundings.

Solutions to Glare Discomfort

If bright lights are deemed to be contributing to discomfort, then they should be removed or their glare reduced in some manner. Many solutions can be implemented inexpensively and without major office redesign.

- Sometimes a single fluorescent luminaire is the source of glare discomfort. The entire fixture can often be turned off by loosening one of the fluorescent tubes. Very often a single offending fixture can be turned off without creating lighting deficiencies because many offices have too much light anyway. When turning off lights, however, consideration must be given to others in the workplace who rely on the light coming from that particular fixture.
- Many offices have two wall switches controlling the fluorescent lights; each controls half of the bulbs in all of the fixtures. Most commonly, both switches are turned on for the day. If the room is brighter than the computer displays, consider turning off half of the lights. Although the first reaction of workers in the area may be negative, longer-term comfort is often improved.
- Some fluorescent light fixtures can be retrofitted with parabolic louvers (the louver is the egg-crate-like cover that directs light into the room). A parabolic louver directs the light from the fluorescent tubes downward in a narrow angle range, hence reducing glare discomfort. Be cautious, however, of louvers that are mirrored as they can actually lead to more glare than what they are designed to reduce.
- The workstation can be reoriented so that bright lights are not in the field of view.
- A very efficient way to eliminate the brightness of overhead fixtures is to wear a visor. Wearing a visor for a day or two can test to determine the extent to which correcting the light problem alleviates discomfort at the end of the day. This can help worker and manager gauge the extent to which glare discomfort is present and the extent to which solutions should be implemented. Wearing the visor can also be an effective permanent solution.
- Avoid bright reflective surfaces. White desktops or floors can reflect excessive amounts of light and serve as sources of glare discomfort. Desktops and other furnishings should have a matte, medium reflective surface. Ceilings should be painted white and walls should be medium light.

- Use blinds or drapes on windows that are sources of glare discomfort. Although most workers appreciate window views, if the window view is considerably brighter than objects in the room (as it almost always is) then the window serves as a source of glare discomfort. Blinds should be adjusted so that workers cannot see the light coming from the window, but the light from the window is directed upward onto the ceiling or sideways so that it is not entering the user's eyes.

- Desk lamps are required if room illumination is inadequate to see critical tasks. However, if improperly located, desk lamps can be sources of glare discomfort. The desk lamp should not direct light directly into the eyes, otherwise it becomes a source of glare discomfort. Also, the desk lamp should not be used to make objects such as reference documents so bright that they exceed recommended luminance levels.

- The brightness of the computer display should be adjusted to match the brightness of the visual objects that immediately surround it.

- Hang or erect partitions. Very often the offending light sources can be eliminated from the field of view by erecting or moving partitions.

Summary

Lighting is often the greatest factor in the work environment causing vision discomfort for computer users. Although the amount of light is important, it is more important to have good light distribution. Good light distribution is accomplished when all of the objects in the field of view have approximately equal brightness. Bright lights or windows are common offending sources and cause discomfort.

References

American National Standard Practice for Office Lighting. New York, New York: American National Standards Institute, Report No.: ANSI/IESNA RP-1-1993.

Berman SM, Greenhouse DS, Bailey IL, Clear RD, Raasch TW. Human electroretinogram responses to video displays, fluorescent lighting, and other high frequency sources. _Optom Vis Sci_ 68(8):645–662, 1991.

Eysel UT BU. Fluorescent tube light evokes flicker responses in visual neurones. _Vis Res_ 24:943–948, 1984.

Guth SK. Prentice memorial lecture: the science of seeing — a search for criteria. _Am J Optom Physiol Opt_, 58(10):870–885, 1981.

Harwood K, Foley P. Temporal resolution: an insight into the video display terminal (VDT) "problem." *Hum Factors* 29(4):447–452,1987.

IES recommended practice for lighting offices containing computer visual display terminals. New York, New York: Illuminating Engineering Society of North America, Report No.: RP-24, 1989.

Laubli T GS, Nishiyama R, Grandjean E. Effects of refresh rates of a simulated CRT display with bright characters on a dark screen. *Int J Ind Ergon* 1:9–20, 1986.

Murata K, Araki S, Kawakami N, Saito Y, Hino E. Central nervous system effects and visual fatigue in VDT workers. *Int Arch Occup Environ Health* 63(2):109–113, 1991.

Sheedy JE, Bailey IL, Raasch TW. Visual acuity and chart luminance. *Am J Optom Physiol Opt* 61(9):595–600, 1984.

Wilkins A. Intermittent illumination from visual display units and fluorescent lighting affects movements of the eyes across text. *Hum Factors* 28(1):75–81, 1986.

Wilkins AJ N-SI, Slater AI, Bedocs L. Fluorescent lighting, headaches and eyestrain. *Lighting Res Technol* 211:11–18, 1989.

Addendum: The Case for Anti-Glare Computer Filters

Sharon Middendorf

CONTENTS

It's an illuminating world — we believe the more light we have, the better it is for us. While it is true that our visual performance improves with light level, it is not always true that more light is better. A paper-intensive environment that needs high ambient light no longer defines the workplace. We have a tale of two worlds in the workplace — paper and electronic information displays. We have computer workplaces that range from manufacturing floors to high-rise offices, from a cozy spot in the home to a seat on a crowded airplane. Addressing the issues of vision, computer displays, and glare in any of these environments can be a challenge, as detailed in previous chapters on computer vision syndrome (Chapter 4) and lighting (Chapter 5).

Why Is Glare on a Computer Display a Problem?

Glare may make us irritable; give us tired, itchy eyes; give us glare-related headaches; and cause us to position our bodies in uncomfortable ways to work around a glare spot — all without our being aware it's happening.

The long-term effects on the visual system when working on a computer, according to the American Optometric Association (AOA) and experts in computer vision syndrome (CVS), may include poor performance on the job, lost time, and aggravation of existing vision conditions. In addition, experts state that CVS may cause an inability to rapidly focus on distance objects.

According to the AOA, people at greatest risk for CVS are computer users who spend three or more hours a day on their computers. In today's electronic office, that could include up to 75% of the computing workforce. That percentage doesn't factor in the personal time people spend on their home computers.

In a study conducted by Cornell University's Ergonomics Laboratory in 1996, direct disability glare was the number one lighting complaint given by cathode ray tube (CRT) computer users. Reflections on an electronic display can affect performance, as was shown in the Cornell study, because it distracts the eye due to its brightness, even though data may still be seen on the display. Light striking the surface of an electronic display can create sharp reflections, with up to 8% of the light reflected back to the user.

In addition, light passing through the display strikes the pixels and reduces contrast by energizing the pixels. The off-state (or black) pixels, are energized or turned on and emit a gray image, conflicting with the on-state pixels and thereby reducing contrast. This is called the signal-to-noise ratio, and contrast reduction occurs when you have greater noise than you have signal. An analogy to contrast reduction on a computer display is having more static

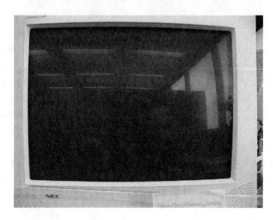

FIGURE 5A.1
Electronic display with reflections.

coming through a radio than you have signal. Unfortunately you can't fine-tune your computer display to get rid of the noise.

What about LCDs?

The influx of liquid crystal displays (LCDs) into the workplace has addressed some of the issues regarding reflections by using a matte surface to diffuse the reflections. The matte surface may be disappearing in the future; the trend in high performance LCDs is back to a glossy surface, reintroducing the problem of reflections on the surface of the display. Whichever surface is used, matte or glossy, users can still experience problems with glare and contrast reduction or image washout. A 2003 survey of LCD users supports this: 39%* reported having a glare problem on the LCD and 85%** of LCD users reacted favorably when an antiglare filter was used with their LCD, stating that they were bothered by glare on their display and preferred working with a glare reduction filter on the display.

What Can Be Done to Reduce or Eliminate Glare on an Electronic Display?

The problem is not how to address the glare and reflections on an electronic computer display; we know several ways to reduce these effects. The problem is that by addressing glare in one area you may create glare in another. A classic example is the duality of the office — higher levels of ambient light are needed for paper-based tasks, which require reflected light for viewing, as opposed to a computer display, which is a self-illuminated device and doesn't require as high a level of ambient light for viewing. Increase the light to accommodate paperwork and you may increase the glare on the computer display, reduce contrast, and create direct disability glare — possibly affecting productivity because of reduced visual performance. Reduce the ambient lighting and you may create a situation that makes it difficult to read printed information. Another problem is that addressing a glare or reflection problem for one person may create similar problems for another person.

---

* n = 2584, +/− 2%
** n = 297, +/− 3%

Lighting

The chapter on lighting is an excellent resource for understanding the overall issues of glare and lighting in the workplace. It includes several suggestions for reducing or eliminating glare on work surfaces and direct glare into your eyes. These include drawing curtains or blinds, changing the overhead lighting, using a visor, and using a task lamp. While most of these will help reduce glare on a computer display, there is a simple and easy-to-use computer accessory that can effectively reduce glare on your display and perhaps minimize the need for expensive architectural or lighting changes. This accessory is known as an anti-glare computer filter.

Anti-Glare Filters

What Are Anti-Glare Filters?

Typically, you will find two types of anti-glare computer filters: anti-reflection (AR) coated glass and anti-reflection coated plastic. In the past, there was a third type of filter, called a mesh filter, which resembled a nylon screen. This product was very effective in diffusing reflections but often caused image degradation due to the crosshatch structure of the mesh; it collected dust and was easily scratched. The AR coated glass and plastic products available today offer a variety of performance levels. It is important to understand what to recommend and to understand the environment in which the computer display is used.

Why Recommend Anti-Glare Filters?

There are four key reasons for recommending anti-glare computer filters:

- The workstation doesn't have to be rearranged to reduce the glare.
- It's an inexpensive solution and may reduce the need for expensive window treatments, lighting, or monitor replacement changes.
- The user gets an immediate solution for instant gratification and relief.
- It doesn't affect the entire office — it addresses the needs of the individual.

How do Anti-Glare Filters Work?

Two optical features are required to provide reflection reduction and contrast improvement — anti-reflection coatings and absorption of transmitted glare.

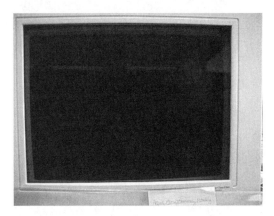

FIGURE 5A.2
Electronic display with anti-glare computer filter.

Anti-Reflection Coatings

The reduction of specular, or mirror, reflections on an electronic display is achieved through multilayer anti-reflection coatings on the front and back surfaces of the glass or plastic. These anti-reflection coatings are three to seven layers of metallized coatings, nearly invisible to the human eye. There is a slight bluish-purple tint (or less common yellow tint) to the filter to indicate the presence of anti-reflection coatings. The coatings use the principle of destructive optical interference to reduce the specular reflections to a level less perceptible to the human eye. Each coating has a slightly different index of refraction, which create phase changes in the light, creating interference waves. Destructive optical interference means that when two light waves of the same frequency and in the same region of space, but out of phase in amplitude combine they cancel, or destroy, each other.

Absorption of Transmitted Glare

In order to minimize contrast loss, it is necessary to add technology that absorbs transmitted glare as it passes through the filter. This is accomplished through one of two means — neutral density colored glass or plastic, or adding a neutral density layer to the anti-reflection coatings. This absorption technology does just that — absorbs the light that transmits through the anti-glare filter, reducing it's overall energy before it passes through the surface

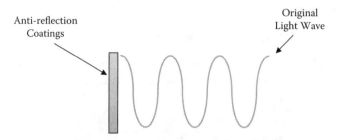

FIGURE 5A.3
Light wave passing through glass with coating.

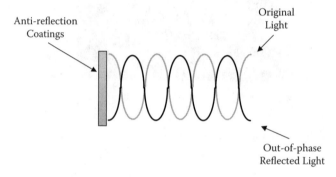

FIGURE 5A.4
Destructive optical interference — waves opposite of each other.

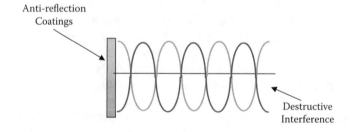

FIGURE 5A.5
Destructive optical interference — waves out of phase neutralize each other.

of the display, thus reducing ability of the light to over-energize the pixels and affect contrast. The light then reflects back from the display, passes through the anti-glare filter once more and is reduced even more in energy, allowing the original image to pass through with higher energy and giving improved contrast. It is actually the dual-absorption technology that is the key to anti-glare computer filters. Critics of anti-glare computer filters often point out that absorption technology reduces the transmission of the original image, making the screen too dark. This may have been the case with the lower transmission anti-glare filters, typically a 31% transmission level. A 31% transmission means that only 31% of the light from the display passes through the anti-glare filter. The anti-glare computer filters available today offer higher transmission levels combined with two-sided anti-reflection coatings — giving the user a product that reduces reflections and improves contrast without compromising transmission of the original image.

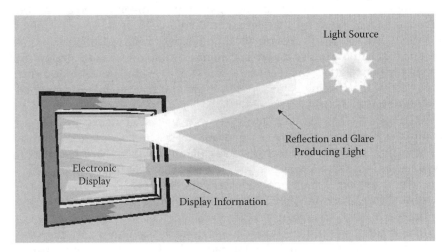

FIGURE 5A.6
Typical reflections off display hide information on screen.

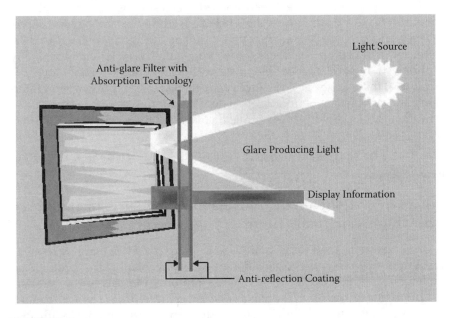

FIGURE 5A.7
Two-sided polarizer reduces glare and allows information on screen to be seen more easily.

What are the Benefits of a Glare-Free or Minimal-Glare Electronic Display?

There are differing opinions on whether or not anti-glare computer filters actually make a difference. Many people feel that changing the lighting, rearranging a workstation, or changing the type of display used can address the problem of glare on the electronic display. All of these are probable solutions, but are not always practical or inexpensive. In addition, care must be taken not to introduce a new ergonomic problem in a workstation rearrangement or to affect the rest of the workforce. Anti-glare computer filters are effective in reducing glare and reflections and have been proven to make a difference for the user.

A 1996 Cornell University study showed that after using an anti-glare computer filter the percentage of problems related to glare-related eye fatigue, tired eyes, trouble focusing eyes, itching/watery eyes, and dry eyes was one half of what it was before using an anti-glare filter. Eighty percent of the users reported the filters reduced glare, making it easier to read their screens. More than one-half said the filters reduced glare and therefore improved their productivity.

Independent, scientific testing of a mid-transmission level anti-glare computer filter to the same international standard that computer monitors must comply with, ISO 9241-7, has shown that this filter can actually improve a monitor's performance against this standard for reflection reduction and contrast improvement. The significance of this testing is that the quality of the anti-reflection coatings and the level of absorption technology are important considerations. There are many products on the market today that claim to be anti-glare computer filters. These filters offer very low quality, if any, anti-reflection performance and little to no absorption technology. It is because of these lower performance products that anti-glare computer filters often are ridiculed by ergonomists when considering options for reducing reflections and glare on an electronic display.

What Features should Be Considered when Recommending an Anti-Glare Computer Filter?

A good feature to look for is an anti-glare computer filter that has received the American Optometric Association's Seal of Acceptance. This product has undergone testing for reflection reduction, uniform transmission, image degradation, and durability. The next way to separate a higher performance anti-glare filter is to look for reflection reduction claims combined with level of transmission. Typical claims to look for would be "up to 99% reflection reduction" and "45 to 55% transmission." A 50% transmission filter offers the best compromise for adequate absorption of transmitted glare to improve contrast while providing a high transmission of the original image. Higher levels of transmission may not reduce transmitted glare enough to adequately improve contrast. Anti-reflection coatings must be on both the front and back surfaces of the filter in order to reduce first surface and total reflections down to a level that will not disturb the user.

Another differentiator to consider is an anti-glare computer filter that has been tested to the same international standards that computer display manufacturers test against for their product — ISO 9241-7. While this standard is designed for computer displays, a computer filter that has been tested with a display against this standard shows that it can help improve a display's performance even more in providing a high level of reflection reduction and contrast enhancement.

It is important to discuss the counter-argument to anti-glare computer filters — that monitors today don't need them because they already have anti-glare treatments. While this is the case for many computer displays, the amount of glare and reflection reduction can be misleading. The trend is going back to glossy displays to give the movie-theater experience for the user. A few key points to keep in mind regarding computer displays and anti-glare treatments:

- Some simply change the state of the reflection from specular to diffuse through silica coatings or etching the surface of the display (a matte finish).
- Some use a spin coating process that may only reduce first surface reflections down about 1 to 2%. Good-quality anti-glare computer filters reduce first surface reflections to less than 1%.
- Flat screens are better, reduce off-axis angle reflections, but still do little for normal incidence reflections.
- Few have absorptive coatings to improve contrast.
- LCDs have many advantages over the older CRT technology, matte surfaces to reduce reflections, but they still have issues with glare and contrast reduction.

Moreover, the trend is going to glossy displays, meaning increased reflections.

Be cautious when selecting an anti-glare filter; make sure it has the science behind its claims. Choose a product from a company whose product quality and integrity you know and trust. If you have questions about the product, call the company or go to their website and find out more. Anti-glare computer filters can be a valuable addition to your tool kit of recommendations for the computing workplace; it's knowing what to look for and what the claims mean that is essential in making the best choice.

References

Allan, T., Glare Screen Home Usage Test Report, Decision Analysis, Inc. study 2003-0559.

Falk, D., Brill, D., Stork, D., *Seeing the Light, Optics in Nature, Photography, Color, Vision and Holography,* John Wiley & Sons, New York, 1986.

Hedge, A., McCrobie, D., Corbet, S., "Reactions to use of a computer screen glare filter," Proceedings of the Human Factors and Ergonomics Society 40th Annual Meeting, 1996.

Howarth, Peter, Lighting in the workplace — a glaring problem?, *The Safety and Health Practitioner, Ergonomics,* supplement, July 1999.

Rancourt, J., Grenawalt, W., Approaches to enhancing VDT viewability and methods of assessing the improvements, *SPIE* Vol. 624 *Advances in Display Technology VI,* 1986.

Sheedy, James E., *Vision at Computer Displays,* Vision Analysis, Walnut Creek, CA, 1995.

6

General Ergonomics Principles

Carolyn M. Sommerich

CONTENTS

Defining Ergonomics

There are a number of well-worded definitions that have been put forth to explain the term *ergonomics*, including this one, slightly modified from Sanders and McCormick (1993):

> Ergonomics discovers and applies information about human behavior, abilities, limitations, and other characteristics to the design of tools, machines, systems, tasks, jobs, and environments for productive, safe, comfortable human use.

Ergonomics promotes and requires a multidisciplinary approach to design, that may draw upon knowledge of biology, anthropology, psychology, engineering, physiology, statistics, occupational medicine, anatomy, industrial design, and optometry, to name several of the relevant disciplines. This multidisciplinary approach is exemplified in this book, which contains chapters on a diverse range of topics, from anatomy and physiology of the eye to the physics of computer monitors.

Before a system is designed, each of the elements must be evaluated, or modified for improvement, although that clearly does not always occur. Ergonomics is often applied reactively, in response to problems that have developed when the human user was not considered during the original design phase of a system or device. Computers provide a good example of this. The first personal computers were units with the display screen directly connected to the keyboard, and eventually to a central processing unit (CPU) also. They were placed on existing office furniture. The result of this was widespread reports of discomfort among users. This eventually resulted in the separation of the display, keyboard, and CPU, and the introduction of adjustable furniture specifically designed to support the various components of the computer at component-specific appropriate heights.

Work systems are made up of more than just the physical components (tools, equipment, workstation, and production materials) with which people work. Other key elements of a work system are the work environment (physical, cultural, and social), work organization (work hours, pay system, assembly line, or other style, etc.), work methods (how the steps in the production process are performed), and tasks performed. The effects of all of these, and how they might interact, should be considered when a system is developed. For example, height adjustability becomes a more important feature for a computer workstation when the computer will be used for extended periods of time by more than one user, and becomes a less important feature if each user only uses the computer for a few minutes during the day. Ergonomists are trained to take a "total view" towards systems design (see Figure 6.1).

Basic Body Mechanics

It is essential to have a basic understanding of the physical construction, physiology, and capabilities of humans in order to design systems, tools, and jobs in which human users will be safe, comfortable, and most productive.

Muscles

Muscle exertion is the basis for all of our physical activities: manipulating small objects in our hands, lifting heavy boxes with our bodies, walking, or positioning ourselves for work at a desk, for example. Muscles are attached to bones via tendons. Muscles contract, and the bones to which they are attached move relative to each other by rotating about the joint that connects

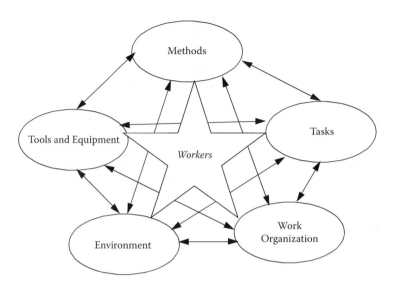

FIGURE 6.1
An ergonomics approach to design means taking a total view of the whole work system, when designing a new system or considering how to improve an existing system.

them. For example, the right index finger flexes to press on the "j" key of a keyboard due to the contraction of the finger flexor muscles. In order to release the "j" key and raise the finger, the finger extensor muscle is activated. This arrangement of muscles, in pairs, is common throughout the body because muscles can only exert contracting forces that pull on bones, yet joints need to move in more than one direction (flex and extend, for example). The muscles that control the elbow are another familiar example of a pair of muscles. The biceps muscle flexes the elbow and the triceps muscle extends the elbow. Generally speaking, neutral joint postures are those positions in which pairs of muscles are in balance when gravity is not a factor.

When the arm is allowed to hang by the side, the wrist is in a neutral position — it is not bent toward the palm or the back of the hand, nor toward the thumb or little finger. Extending the wrist, while the arm is at the side, requires contraction of the wrist extensor muscles. When the hands float above the keyboard when typing, the wrist extensor muscles are also active, even if the wrist is in a neutral position. This is because gravity exerts a downward force on the hand when the forearm is positioned horizontally. The wrist tends to flex due to the pull of gravity on the hand. In order to keep the wrist straight, the wrist extensor muscles must contract to counteract the gravitational force on the hands. Holding such a position becomes uncomfortable after a time. This is because the muscles are being asked to exert force continuously, which does not allow them to operate in their most efficient manner. Blood flows best through muscles as they alternate between contraction and relaxation. Blood flow within a muscle may be impeded during sustained contractions. Because blood flow is a key element in the metabolic process (the means by which energy is transferred from the foods we eat to chemicals and energy muscles use to function), if the blood flow is reduced, then eventually the muscle will fatigue. Muscle fatigue is associated with discomfort and reduction in the ability to control the muscle (e.g., to position a limb precisely where desired or exert a specific desired amount of force). Fatigue effects can be short or long term, depending on the pattern of development (one-time event or prolonged or repeated development). Long-term effects can include damage or destruction of some of the individual muscle fibers that make up a muscle. External supports, such as the seatpan of a chair, forearm supports, and back rest, have been shown to be effective in alleviating fatigue and reducing discomfort in workers.

Ergonomic Design Principles

Several ergonomic design principles stem from what we know about how muscles function, and these will be utilized to explain some other key, basic body mechanics concepts. These have been modified from Sjøgaard (1999):

- Design the work system to allow for variation in work postures.
- Design the work system based on principles of optimization of workload.
- Design the work system such that employees perform a variety of different tasks.

Design the work system to allow for variation in work postures. These may center on neutral postures, but sustaining any posture for an extended period of time is not good for muscles or other body components. Postures may be maintained by internal supports (muscles), external supports (chair, arm rest, etc.), or some combination of these. Problems with sustained support from muscles were addressed just above. Problems with sustained support from external sources include joint stiffness and compression of passive soft tissue. A common site of soft tissue compression is the skin and the layers of soft tissue between the skin and the ischial tuberosities (sitting bones), which is associated with sitting for long periods of time. Another is the cubital tunnel ("funny bone" region at the elbow) through which an important nerve passes, which can be compressed when the elbows are rested upon for an extended period of time.

Neutral joint postures are generally preferred over nonneutral postures for several reasons. Muscles change length when the joint with which they are associated changes position. For example, when the wrist is extended, the wrist extensor muscles are shortened, and when the wrist is flexed the extensor muscles must lengthen. However, muscles can produce the most force when they are at their neutral length. So if a task required 15% of a muscle's strength when it was at its neutral length, that same task would require a greater percentage of the muscle's strength if the muscle were shortened when called upon to perform the same task. Another reason for preferring neutral joint positions is that soft tissue in the area of the joint can be compressed when joints are positioned away from neutral. Two important and common examples of this are seen in computer users. Many people type with their wrists in an extended position. From a number of research studies, we know that an important nerve that runs through the forearm and into the hand (the median nerve) can be compressed rather severely at the wrist when the wrist is extended or flexed more than about 30 degrees. This can lead to problems with the functioning of the nerve, and potentially could contribute to the development of carpal tunnel syndrome. Another common area of discomfort in computer users is the shoulder. Shoulder discomfort can develop as a consequence of working with a computer mouse that is located some distance from the keyboard. Raising the arm even modestly (30 to 45 degrees away from the body, in front or to the side) elevates the pressure within the muscle that helps to raise the arm (supraspinatus muscle). The consequence of this is reduced blood flow in both the muscle and its tendon. Another problem for the supraspinatus tendon when the arm is raised is that it can be compressed between the humerus (upper arm bone) and the acromion (a boney process that is the outermost point of the scapula), which can lead to development of tendinitis.

One way to facilitate variation in work posture is to provide adjustable furniture, and instruction on how it is to be used. Instruction is key, because what is taught is that the furniture is not to be adjusted once for the user and never again. One of the benefits of adjustable furniture is that users can adjust it throughout the day to facilitate changes in their posture. Sit/stand workstations are particularly useful in this regard.

Design the work system based on principles of optimization of workload. It was mentioned earlier that neutral joint positions are preferred over non-neutral postures, but that variation in posture is also important. This is part of the concept that is introduced through the term optimization in this design principle. Ergonomic design is not about finding the one best posture or the method that requires the very least amount of muscular effort, but about optimizing the work system, which means removing extreme exposures (in effort, posture, etc.) to the greatest extent possible, but then affording a mixed exposure that taxes operators to an extent that is safe and healthy, and allows for the greatest productivity under those circumstances. With a few exceptions (such as exposure to vibration or contact stress), most exposure curves are U-shaped. That is, either too much or too little is a problem. Too much motion is bad, as is too little. Too much force required to be exerted is bad, as is the need for no force. A job that poses little mental challenge is as bad as one that is always excessively challenging. Optimizing workload means providing a healthy range of exposures/demands, both physical and cognitive.

Design the work system such that employees perform a variety of different tasks. The idea here is to help provide that variety in posture, muscle force activation, and cognitive workload, in part, by creating jobs that consist of a variety of tasks. What is key to this principle is the ability to recognize when tasks are different and when they are not. For example, a word processing task and a task requiring a Web-based literature search are not sufficiently different when considering the postures, physical loads, and physical activity required, though they do provide different levels of cognitive load. If one of the tasks also required walking to a library or printer to retrieve some of the items identified in the literature search, that would begin to add variety in the physical demands, also.

Though visual considerations on the job have not been mentioned yet, in the remaining sections of this chapter, the reader will see that these ergonomic design principles are also appropriate for eye health and safety as well.

Work-Related Visual Strain

Workers in many different lines of work experience work-related visual strain (asthenopia or discomfort), including welders, those working in the electronics industry, and those who work with microscopes. Any job that requires intense visual concentration is likely to be associated with visual strain in workers. By far, the greatest number of reports written about visual strain (discomfort) concern computer users. Based on these reports, visual strain appears to be common in workers who use computers on the job. For example, in a study of desktop and notebook computer-using professionals, Sommerich (2002) found that eye discomfort was the most common body part location of discomfort in the respondents. Seventy-six percent of study participants experienced eye discomfort in the 12 months preceding the study; 68% of those who experienced eye discomfort found that on-the-job activities made their eye discomfort worse. Twenty percent of the respondents reported experiencing eye discomfort frequently (i.e., "quite often" or "almost always") when using a computer. As with other types of discomfort, and as commonly observed in studies of occupational discomfort, female respondents were more likely to report eye discomfort than were the male respondents.

Visual strain in computer users has been attributed to a number of factors, including weekly time spent using computers (Rechichi et al., 1996), computer display location and orientation (Bergqvist and Knave, 1994), inappropriate lighting and glare, other environmental factors (such as dust or dry air), and personal factors (including uncorrected visual problems) (Cole, 2003), though the latter three are not unique to workers who use computers. The surface of the eye can be affected by environmental factors, and the amount of surface that is exposed can be affected by the location of the object being viewed (when eyes look downward, less ocular surface area is exposed to the environment because the eyelids are drawn down with the downward rotation of the eyeball). Other components of the eye that are points of concern are the muscles within and outside of the eyeball, because these muscles can be strained by some work conditions. The ciliary muscles within the eyeball contract to allow the lens to become more rounded for viewing near objects. These can be strained if a person continuously looks at near objects and does not vary his/her gaze to look at more distant objects from time to time. These muscles can also be strained as a result of viewing poor quality or very small text. There are two sets of small muscles in the iris that react to lighting conditions and may be strained as a result of working under adverse lighting conditions. In low light conditions, the radial muscle fibers of the iris contract to dilate the pupil, while in bright light the circular muscle fibers of the iris contract to constrict the pupil. Additionally, the extraocular muscles, muscles that are outside of the eyeball and whose job it is to position the eyeball, can become fatigued when their activity is not allowed to vary, which occurs when the location of the visual target does not change, particularly when viewing targets in difficult locations (such as visual targets that are near and positioned high (eye level or above)). Viewing near objects at a high level (e.g., eye-level) puts a strain on the extraocular muscles, because the muscles that rotate the eyeball up, due to where they attach to the eyeball, also tend to rotate the eyeball laterally (outward). By contrast, the extraocular muscles that rotate the eyeball down also tend to rotate the eye inward. As such, converging both eyes to focus upon a high, near target can put a strain on those extraocular muscles.

It is easy to see that the three ergonomic design principles listed in the previous section need to be followed in order to minimize work-related visual strain. *Variation in work posture applied to the eyes* can be thought of as designing work such that a person's gaze is directed in various locations (angles and distances) throughout the day, which would vary the position of the eyeball during the day so as to not strain the ocular muscles. *Optimization of workload applied to the eyes* would mean that visual targets and lighting conditions are in recommended ranges, such that all of the muscles of the eye are worked to some extent during the day, but none are overworked. *Performing a variety of tasks* should ensure that viewing distances, viewing angles, and visual targets change throughout the day, again, in order that none of the muscles of the eyes are overworked. Additionally, because blink rates vary with different tasks (e.g., people tend to blink less frequently when viewing a computer monitor), the ocular surface will be better protected if a variety of tasks are performed during the workday.

Viewing Distance and Angles

Quite a bit of research has been conducted to identify appropriate viewing distances and angles, particularly with respect to viewing computer monitors. This has occurred because of the high prevalence of visual discomfort

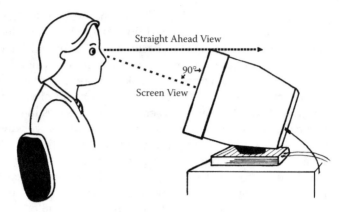

FIGURE 6.2
Depiction of gaze angle defined relative to horizontal.

that is associated with computer use, as well as a high prevalence of musculo-skeletal discomfort, particularly neck discomfort. It has also occurred because, unlike books or paper, users cannot easily reposition their computer monitors (due to the weight of the monitor, limited room on the desktop for positioning the monitor, and common use of desks that are not height-adjustable), so companies that have an interest in ergonomics have the desire to set up workstations for their employees that will allow them to be both comfortable and productive. Psihogios et al. (2001) reviewed many studies on viewing angle preference, musculoskeletal strain as a function of computer monitor location, and studies that defined neutral posture. They also conducted studies on these topics, themselves (Psihogios et al., 2001; Sommerich et al., 2001; Turville et al., 1998). Based on their own studies and those of other researchers, Psihogios et al. (2001) concluded that a mid-level monitor location was likely to provide the best compromise to minimize both visual and musculoskeletal strain associated with computer use, for most users. Mid-level placement refers to a gaze angle of 10 to 17.5 degrees to the center of the monitor, relative to horizontal (see Figure 6.2). However, they also suggested that "individual differences in visual capabilities (such as the use of bifocals), physical make-up, work tasks, and other workstation design elements signal that fine-tuning of placement" may be needed to meet some users' needs.

Several standards also provide recommendations for computer monitor location. These are presented in Table 6.1.

Interaction of Body Posture and Visual Task Requirements

A number of studies of computer monitor placement have shown that head and neck posture, and sometimes trunk posture as well, are directly affected

TABLE 6.1

Recommendations for Computer Monitor Locations, from Some National and International Standards

Standard	Distance	Vertical Angle	Horizontal Angle
Australian Standard (AS, 1990)	35 to 75 cm for the primary display	15 to 45 degrees downward from horizontal, eye-level gaze; refers to this angle as "optimal"	Within 15 degrees on either side of the centerline of the viewer, for the primary display
International Standards Organization (ISO, 1992)	At least 40 cm, and is dependent upon the size of the characters	0 to 60 degrees downward from horizontal, eye-level gaze; "preferred" is 20 to 22 degrees downward	
BSR/HFES (BSR/HFES, 2002) (This is the revision of ANSI/HFS 100-1988.)	50 to 100 cm	0 to 60 degrees downward from horizontal, eye-level gaze; center at 15 to 20 degrees downward	Within 17.5 degrees on either side of the centerline of the viewer

by the location of the computer monitor. When a computer monitor is placed higher, users assume more upright head, neck, and trunk postures. When a computer monitor is placed in a lower location, users tend to rotate the head forward, flex the neck forward, and flex the trunk forward or round the back (hunch over). Eye position also changes as a function of monitor location, with eyes rotating upward or downward in response to raising or lowering the monitor. The concern for the development of musculoskeletal discomfort in computer users arises when the head, neck, and trunk are noticeably flexed forward, because it requires more muscular effort to maintain these postures than to sit more upright. When upright, the head is naturally balanced over the spine (requiring little muscle activity to maintain the position), and the back is in contact with (and supported by) the backrest of the chair. As mentioned previously, it is important to design a workstation so as to minimize both musculoskeletal and visual strain. So, placement of the monitor such that the center is 10 to 20 degrees below the horizontal is suggested as a starting point.

It has also been shown that, when using a notebook computer, the flexed body posture becomes more acute as the size of the computer becomes smaller (Villanueva et al., 1998). This is likely to be due to the user's perception of a need to access a smaller visual target, as well as a smaller target for the hands. It is suggested that notebook computers be used as standalone units only when away from an office setting, and only for short work periods. When used in an office setting, notebook PCs should be connected to peripheral devices (a mouse or other external pointing device and external keyboard, at a minimum) in order to allow the user to adopt more comfortable postures and allow for more variation in postures. More information regarding notebook computer use is provided in a separate section, toward the end of this chapter.

Another case of visual needs driving body posture is seen among bifocal wearers. They tend to either extend the neck and rotate the head back or adopt a "forward head posture" (flexed neck plus positioning of the head in front of the neck and trunk with the chin jutting out in front). These postures are adopted when the computer user attempts to view a computer monitor located at desktop height or above through his/her bifocals. The strength and position of the bifocal (at the bottom of the lens) were based upon the need to view near objects in low locations, and as such are not an appropriate solution for viewing a computer monitor (an object at a middle distance that is usually located in a mid- to eye-level location). Although some computer furniture is designed to position the monitor low (submerged below the desk surface), this also means the monitor will not be positioned near (the other location factor relevant to bifocal use). Another problem with locating the monitor below the desktop is that there is then less room under the desk for the legs to be comfortably positioned. In the next section, more workstation options are discussed.

Computer Workstation Options

The basic components needed for tailoring a workstation to a user are a stable, adjustable height chair and a desktop of sufficient depth. Narrow desktops limit the distance the computer monitor can be placed away from the user. Studies have shown that computer users tend to prefer to view monitors at distances of 70 to 90 cm (Jaschinski et al., 1998; Sommerich et al., 1998). As CRT-style computer monitors increased in screen size, they also increased in depth, making it more difficult to achieve these desired distances. One option for achieving this distance is to place the monitor in a corner. In all cases, though, the user should always be able to position himself/herself directly in front of the monitor and the keyboard (see Figure 6.3). The use of flat panel displays makes it easier to achieve the desired distance between the monitor and the user on smaller desktop surfaces. Placing the monitor directly on the desktop surface, and then adjusting the height of the chair so that the top of the display and the user's eye are at a similar height usually ensures the preferred viewing angle of 10 to 20 degrees below eye level to the center of the monitor. After adjusting the chair height, the user's feet should be able to be placed flat on the floor so that the feet do not dangle (which would indicate the seatpan is too high); conversely

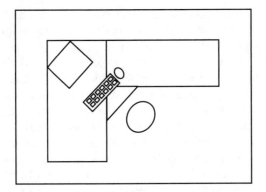

FIGURE 6.3
Bird's eye view of a corner arrangement of a computer workstation that affords a greater distance between the computer monitor and the user. Note that the keyboard, monitor and user are all aligned. The other advantage this arrangement affords is the support of the arms on the work surface when the user types on the keyboard or uses the mouse.

the knees should not be higher than the hips (which would indicate the seatpan is too low). If the seatpan is too high, a footrest can be incorporated. If the seatpan is too low, the work surface should be raised.

Regardless of how well-tuned the workstation is to the user, it is still important for the user to vary his/her posture throughout the day. This includes making adjustments to the chair height and other adjustments that may be built into the chair, as well as getting up from the chair periodically. Sit/stand workstations afford users the opportunity to perform their desk-based work in a wider range of postures than does a traditional seated workstation option. Users can alternate between sitting and standing to work, but can also vary the height of the work surface somewhat while sitting or standing, thus providing additional variation in work posture throughout the day.

A Few Notes on Notebook Computer Use

In 1975 there were fewer than 200,000 computers in the United States (Juliussen and Petska-Juliussen, 1994). By contrast, U.S. PC shipments for 2004 were expected to number 56 million units; worldwide shipments were expected to number around 165 million units (Spooner, 2003). By 2007, notebook computers (NPC) are expected to constitute 40% of worldwide shipments and 47% of U.S. shipments; in 2004 they were expected to be 30 and 34% of those shipments, respectively (Spooner, 2004). The growing use of notebook computers raises concerns for development of discomfort in their users, as have some recent reports on student NPC users (Harris and Straker, 2000) and adult workers who use NPCs (Heasman et al., 2000; Sommerich, 2002).

In brief, from a physical ergonomics perspective, the design of NPCs is a step backward, in that, once again, the keyboard and the monitor are joined so as to not permit independent location of each of these components. This means that either the user's hands and arms can be positioned comfortably or the head and neck can be. Comfortable positioning of the whole body cannot be achieved without the use of peripheral devices (external keyboard, monitor, or pointing device). When used in a stand-alone configuration, users tend to position a notebook computer to favor the arms and shoulders, by choosing to place the computer at a height that is comfortable for typing (Straker et al., 1997). As a result, users must angle the head and neck downward to view the NPC's built-in monitor. However, there is evidence to suggest that users are more comfortable (Berkhout et al., 2004; Price and Dowell, 1998; Sommerich, 2002), display more variation in posture (Sommerich et al., 2002), and are more productive (Berkhout et al., 2004; Sommerich, 2002) when NPCs are not used in a stand-alone configuration. In an office setting, simple pedestal-type stands or newer stand designs that incorporate a document holder into their design (Berkhout et al., 2004) can be used to elevate the NPC above the desktop, to afford a more comfortable viewing angle for the user, as could something as simple as a telephone book. An external pointing device and keyboard are inexpensive options that complete the setup. An external mouse can easily be stowed in a computer carrying case, so that this peripheral device can be utilized most places that the computer is used outside of an office setting, as well.

Summary

In this chapter, we have provided some basic concepts and suggestions for working more comfortably and productively with computers. It is essential to have a good physical work set up, but the way in which someone works will also have a major influence on his/her comfort. Variation in work tasks and postures has been emphasized throughout this chapter. Taking breaks from work is another form of variation. Taking short breaks of 5 min or so every hour, in addition to traditional 15 min morning and afternoon breaks and a break for lunch, has been shown to decrease discomfort (eye and musculoskeletal) while not impeding productivity (Galinsky et al., 2000), which are the primary goals of ergonomic design, as defined at the beginning of this chapter.

References

AS 1990, Screen-based workstations, part 2: Workstation furniture, AS 3590.2-1990, Standards Australia.

Bergqvist, U.O. and Knave, B.G. 1994, Eye discomfort and work with visual display terminals, *Scandinavian Journal of Work, Environment, and Health*, 20, 27–33.

Berkhout, A.L., Hendriksson-Larsen, K. and Bongers, P. 2004, The effect of using a laptop station compared to using a standard laptop pc on the cervical spine torque, perceived strain and productivity, *Applied Ergonomics*, 35, 147–152.

BSR/HFES 2002, Human factors engineering of computer workstations, BSR/HFES100 — Draft Standard for Trial Use, The Human Factors and Ergonomics Society.

Cole, B.L. 2003, Do video display units cause visual problems? — a bedside story about the processes of public health decision-making, *Clinical and Experimental Optometry*, 86, 205–220.

Galinsky, T.L., Swanson, N.G., Sauter, S.L., Hurrell, J.J., and Schleifer. 2000, A field study of supplementary rest breaks for data-entry operators, *Ergonomics*, 43, 622–638.

Harris, C. and Straker, L. 2000, Survey of physical ergonomics issues associated with school childrens' use of laptop computers, *International Journal of Industrial Ergonomics*, 26, 337–346.

Heasman, T., Brooks, A. and Stewart, T. 2000, Health and safety of portable display screen equipment, 304/2000, Health & Safety Executive, United Kingdom.

ISO 1992, Ergonomic requirements for office work with visual display terminals (VDTs) — workplace requirements, ISO 9241-3, International Standards Organization.

Jaschinski, W., Heuer, H. and Kylian, H. 1998, Preferred position of visual displays relative to the eyes: A field study of visual strain and individual differences, *Ergonomics*, 41, 1034–1049.

Juliussen, E. and Petska-Juliussen, K. 1994, *7th Annual Computer Industry Almanac*. (Austin: Computer Industry Almanac, Inc.).

Price, J.A. and Dowell, W.R. 1998, Laptop configurations in offices: Effects on posture and discomfort, *Proceedings of Human Factors and Ergonomics Society 42nd Annual Meeting*, Chicago, 629–633.

Psihogios, J.P., Sommerich, C.M., Mirka, G.M., and Moon, S.D. 2001, A field evaluation of monitor placement effects in VDT users, *Applied Ergonomics*, 32, 313–325.

Reichichi, C., De Moja, C.A., and Scullica, L. 1996, Psychology of computer use: XXXVI. Visual discomfort and different types of work at videodisplay terminals, *Perceptual and Motor Skills*, 82, 935–938.

Sanders, M.S. and McCormick, E.J. 1993, *Human Factors in Engineering and Design* 7th ed. (New York: McGraw-Hill).

Sjøgaard, G. 1999. Low-level static exertions, in W. Karwowski and Marras, W. (eds.), *The Occupational Ergonomics Handbook* (Boca Raton: CRC Press). 247–259.

Sommerich, C.M. 2002, A survey of desktop and notebook computer use by professionals, *Proceedings of Human Factors and Ergonomics Society 46th Annual Meeting*, in Baltimore, MD: Human Factors and Ergonomics Society.

Sommerich, C.M., Joines, S. M.B., and Psihogios, J.P. 1998, Effects of VDT viewing angle on user biomechanics, comfort, and preference, *Proceedings of 42nd Annual Meeting of the Human Factors and Ergonomics Society,* in Chicago: The Human Factors and Ergonomics Society.

Sommerich, C.M., Joines, S.M.B., and Psihogios, J.P. 2001, Effects of computer monitor viewing angle and related factors on strain, performance, and preference outcomes, *Human Factors,* 43, 39–55.

Sommerich, C.M., Starr, H., Smith, C.A., and Shivers, C. 2002, Effects of notebook computer configuration and task on user biomechanics, productivity, and comfort, *International Journal of Industrial Ergonomics,* 30, 7–31.

Spooner, J.G. 2003, IDC rethinks PC forecast, CNET News.com, http://news.zdnet.co.uk/hardware/0,39020351,39116143,00.htm.

Spooner, J.G. 2004, Consumers keep notebook sales on a roll, CNET News.com, http://www.cnet.com/4520-6018_1-105833.html.

Straker, L., Jones, K.J., and Miller, J. 1997, A comparison of the postures assumed when using laptop computers and desktop computers, *Applied Ergonomics,* 28, 263–268.

Turville, K.L., Psihogios, J.P., Ulmer, T.R., and Mirka, G.A. 1998, The effects of video display terminal height on the operator: A comparison of the 15 degree and 40 degree recommendations, *Applied Ergonomics,* 29, 239–246.

Villanueva, M.B., Jonai, H., and Saito, S. 1998, Ergonomic aspects of portable personal computers with flat panel displays (pc-fpds): Evaluation of posture, muscle activities, discomfort, and performance, *Industrial Health,* 36, 282–289.

7

Vision Examinations and Glasses

Stephen Glasser

CONTENTS

Introduction

A vision examination by the appropriate eye care professional is more than an examination of the eyes. It is an examination of the individual's visual system as well. The visual system starts with the eyes, continues through the optic nerves to the lower centers of the brain, and eventually to the back of the visual cortex in the brain. This is where visual perception begins. Through a series of tests, the doctor is able to evaluate not only the health of the eyes, but to determine any necessary optical correction and the visual efficiency of the patient.

Computer use brings with it unique visual demands. Only through a comprehensive visual examination can the doctor determine if the capabilities of the individual suffice for the demands of the work environment.

The purpose of this chapter is not to teach the examination methods, but to allow the reader to understand the components that make up a complete evaluation of the eyes and visual system.

The Eye Care Professionals

Optometrist (OD)

An optometrist is a doctor of optometry who, following four years of undergraduate studies, completes four additional years of specialized training in a school of optometry. These specialized studies include instruction in vision and eye examination, as well as the detection and treatment of eye infections and diseases. Of note is that optometrists are uniquely trained in the areas of visual coordination, contact lenses, the optics of eyeglasses, visual efficiency, subnormal vision, and the development of vision.

Ophthalmologist (MD)

An ophthalmologist is a doctor of medicine who, following four years of undergraduate studies, completes four years of medical school. After completion, the physician serves one year of internship and three or more years of specialized medical and surgical training in the field of eye care. Of note is that the ophthalmologist is uniquely trained in the areas of surgical techniques and treatment of eye diseases.

Optician

An optician is a technician who is trained to fill the eyewear prescriptions of optometrists and ophthalmologists. Most states require formal education and licensing of opticians; a few allow for apprenticeships. An optician fabricates lenses, fitting them into eyeglass frames and adjusts these frames to fit the wearer. Some states allow opticians to fit contact lenses.

The Examination

It is not the purpose of this chapter to explain every component of the visual examination. However, it is important that those who hear the complaints and problems of employees understand what is involved in a thorough examination and the reporting of the results.

The examination of an individual's vision is made up of two main components. The first component is a series of tests to determine the health and condition of various structures of the eyes. The second component of the vision examination is that of visual function. It is this testing of visual function that determines how well the eyes will function in their everyday environment.

To most people, perhaps the most familiar vision term is 20/20. From a scientific standpoint, it indicates that an individual is capable of seeing a letter that subtends 20 min of arc at a distance of 20 ft. In practical terms, this means that from a distance of 20 ft an individual is capable of seeing the average smallest letter physically able to be recognized at that distance. This is a designation of acuity, or sharpness of vision.

Most people are able to gauge their acuity. With few exceptions, most individuals can determine whether they are able to read both for distance and near objects clearly. The same cannot be said of visual function. Visual function is defined as the efficient and coordinated working of the eyes with each other.

Let's take an example. An office worker is swamped with computer tasks. This requires him to focus on the computer for extended periods of time. His last eye examination showed that he is seeing 20/20 with each eye, for both distance and near. However, he is now complaining of problems keeping the computer screen clear and finds that he is tiring much more quickly than before. Excluding any other physical causes, this worker has problems with his visual function. Because of the extended near-point work, this worker must maintain a rather constant focus at the computer distance. While this may be easy for short periods of time, extended periods can cause symptoms. An analogy would be holding a brick out at arms length. It's easy at first, but as time passes, the muscles start to fatigue and the task becomes much more difficult, if not impossible. The same can be said of the eyes. Extended close work causes the focusing system of the eyes to work without rest. While acuity may or may not remain fine, the function of maintaining that focusing ability easily becomes the problem.

Situations like this are not uncommon. The vast majority of computer users have visual symptoms (which are now commonly referred to as computer vision syndrome, see Chapter 4), which may erroneously be attributed to conditions such as boredom, stress, and poor eating habits, to name a few. While these are certainly possibilities, the most likely problem lies with the eyes.

Components of the Standard Examination

History

A good eye examination always begins with a good history. It is important that the patient be frank and honest with the doctor as to any problems, both visual and otherwise, that are being experienced. In many cases, symptoms and complaints that may seem at first glance to be independent of the visual system are, in fact, related.

Physical Evaluation

The eyes are examined both externally and internally to ensure that their health is maintained. The eyes are the only place in the body where internal blood vessels are visible without surgery. The eyes are checked for such vision-threatening conditions as glaucoma, cataracts, and macular degeneration. In addition, the eyes are checked for changes due to such systemic diseases as hypertension, diabetes, and HIV-AIDS. This evaluation is not only an examination of the eyes, but of the body as well.

Visual Acuity

In the course of the examination, visual acuities are taken. Set at the standard of 20/20, this measures the sharpness of one's vision at a far viewing distance. Acuity is also measured at a near reading distance, usually 16 in. While this had traditionally been the only near viewing distance tested, many doctors are starting to look at the "intermediate" viewing distance as well. This is the distance at which the computer display is viewed. This is why it is critical to tell the doctor the exact computer viewing distance, if possible.

Entrance Tests

Depending upon the needs and age of the patient, tests are performed to evaluate for color perception, depth perception, eye alignment, and smoothness of eye movement. These tests are the preliminary part of testing visual function.

Prescription Determination

Also known as the refraction, this part consists of a series of tests to determine whether the patient is nearsighted, farsighted, or has astigmatism .

Visual Function and Facility Testing

As discussed previously, this area of testing may be the most important aspect of testing for the vocational well-being of the worker. It is here that the individual's visual efficiency is determined. Measurements that show strain, stress, or inability to adapt to the visual environment may lead the patient to have problems in the workplace.

Summation

This component allows the doctor to explain the findings of the examination to the patient. In addition, recommendations as to the best methods of care are presented. These recommendations may be as simple as a new prescription for contact lenses or glasses, or may indicate that further testing is necessary, including a full ergonomic visual evaluation.

Ergonomic Visual Evaluation

An ergonomic visual evaluation is composed of a series of tests and observations that are made specific to the patient's working environment. This evaluation may be conducted in the optometric office, in the workplace, or a combination of both.

While many patients have their problems solved through the standard examination, many cannot. Due to individual office ergonomic setups, many patients require examination techniques that go beyond the standard testing. These may include an expanded history; measuring focusing ability over time, known as accommodative facility testing; and testing the tear quality.

In addition, the conditions under which the individual is working may also need to be examined. Office lighting, glare sources, postural evaluation, and working distances are but a few of the measurements that may be necessary in order to determine the individual's needs. Depending upon the doctor's expertise, knowledge, and instrumentation available, these determinations may be made in a number of ways. Patient questionnaires, site visits, and environmental photographs are some of the methods that may help the doctor make the correct ergonomic and visual correction recommendations.

Computer Vision Screening

Recently, a new method for screening computer users has been introduced. It is a software program run on the user's computer that consists of a series of visual acuity and function tests. Unlike the methods described previously, this new method of testing is the first that allows patients to be tested in the computer-using environments in which they work.

Computer Eyewear

Eyeglasses

Most prescribed eyeglasses are for general purposes — driving, movies, TV, shopping, etc., allowing the wearer to perform a variety of tasks. However, there are also specifically designed lenses that are made to allow the wearer to perform specific tasks more easily. "Computer glasses" are designed with these types of lenses.

A computer prescription is any lens that allows the wearer to see the computer and the surrounding environment clearly and more comfortably. They do not, however, necessarily allow clear vision for other tasks and distances. The following discussion will look at some of the more popular computer-use lenses available and their appropriate applications and limitations.

Single Vision

Single vision lenses, as the name implies, are lenses that have a single prescription fabricated in them. This allows for a range of visual clarity and comfort. For some individuals, this range may extend from very close to very far away. However, as one gets older or has greater visual demands, such as computer use, the range of clarity and comfort may become smaller.

For example, an elderly individual can have single vision lenses that would allow them to drive and see distances clearly. However, the person's near

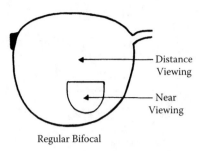

Regular Bifocal

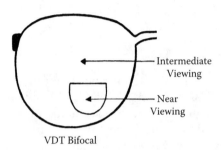

VDT Bifocal

FIGURE 7.1
Typical and task-specific types of bifocals.

vision, for reading, would be blurred. A second pair of single vision lenses may allow for clear and comfortable reading. However, the person's distance vision would then be blurred.

For computer users, it is important to not only have clarity at the distance they are working from, but comfort as well. For this reason, it is important that the patient inform the doctor of the distance from the eye to computer screen, the keyboard, hard copy, etc., so that the doctor can determine whether there is an indication for different prescriptions at these varying distances. Single vision lenses that allow the individual to read the computer screen but do not relieve the strain on the eyes from prolonged near focusing are neither beneficial nor efficient.

Intermediate/Near Bifocals

Conventional multi-focal lenses are designed so that the upper portion of the lens contains the distance prescription while the lower portion of the lens contains the near prescription. However, the lenses can be changed by the doctor, so that the upper portion of the lens contains the intermediate, or computer screen prescription, while the lower portion of the lens continues to contain the near, or keyboard and mouse prescription (Figure 7.1). This design can be effective, however it is limited by its range (only two prescription areas) and the disconcerting nature of a lens that contains a line through the middle of the viewing area (the bifocal line).

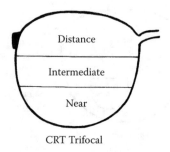

CRT Trifocal

FIGURE 7.2
Early "CRT" trifocal lens with three viewing distance zones.

Computer Trifocals

To take computer bifocals one step further, computer trifocals were developed in the late 1970s. As with the bifocals, lined segments of the lens separate the distance prescription area at the top of the lens from the computer screen prescription in the center of the lens, and from the reading prescription at the bottom of the lens (Figure 7.2).

As with the computer bifocal design, there is no smooth transition between the viewing areas of the lens. In addition, the increased weight of the lens often made continual wear difficult.

Progressive Addition Lenses

In the later part of the 1970s, a new design of lens was refined. Unlike previous eyeglass lenses that required lines on the lens to separate the distance and near areas, this new design allowed for a gradual change in the power of the lens, from the top distance prescription to the bottom reading prescription. This eliminated the appearance of the lines on the lens while allowing the wearer to see clearly at all distances. However, in order to accommodate this gradual change in prescription, the wearer had to look down the center of the lens to achieve the sharpest vision. As the wearer's gaze went off to one side or the other, distortions appeared and increased as the gaze went further away from that centerline. New manufacturing methods now allow the range of clear undistorted vision to be expanded, but not eliminated. In general, a standard progressive lens is not recommended for a full-time computer user. The intermediate zone (designed for the computer viewing distance) is too narrow to view the entire screen without head movement, thus creating a visually disturbing situation.

With the increasing use of computers in the workplace, progressive lens manufacturers have turned their development to the design of eyeglass lenses that would correct the vision of the computer user. Their purpose is to give the entire work area a clear view without creating a need for excessive head movements. These designs are given work-related names, such as Technica, Desktop, Office, On-line, Business, Browser, and Access.

The designs do vary. The Technica lens, for example, has a very large reading area at the bottom of the lens, a slightly smaller intermediate viewing area at the center of the lens, and a very small distance area at the top of the lens. The Access lens has a very large reading area covering the entire lower part of the lens, and an equally large intermediate area covering the entire upper part of the lens. This second design provides the largest usable viewing areas of the lens with the least amount of distortion.

The determination of which design is right for the individual can only be achieved through a thorough vision examination and discussion of work habits and environment with the employee's eye care provider.

Lens Tints

When computers were first introduced into the workplace, eye care professionals postulated that the screen colors would appear sharper with a light tinting of the eyeglass lenses of the computer user. At that time, there were three primary computer screen colors in use: green letters, amber letters, or white letters — all on a black background. Using various theories of light behavior and optical physics, it was determined that a person using green letters would benefit from a light magenta tint, a person using amber letters would benefit from a blue tint, and a person using white letters would benefit from a neutral gray tint. While the theories behind the use of lens colors may have been sound, the actual benefits to the computer user have now been disproved. In addition, with the advent of multicolored screens, the concept of lens tints based on screen color has become obsolete.

With this being said, there is some evidence that a light rose (or pink) colored tint is of benefit to most computer users. The reasoning behind this recommendation is the fact that most offices tend to be illuminated with fluorescent lighting, which tends to emit light wavelengths more heavily in the blue end of the spectrum. The light rose tinting of the eyeglass lenses tends to mute this overexposure and allows for a more relaxed visual environment. See Chapter 5 for more details on the lighting aspects of the computer environment.

Anti-Reflective Coatings

Light transmitted through a normal eyeglass lens only allows 92% of the light to pass completely through it; 4% is reflected by the front surface of the lens, while an additional 4% is reflected by the back surface. However, a coating can be applied to the surfaces of the lens that effectively cancels out this reflection and allows 99% of the light to pass through.

This has a double benefit to the eyeglass wearer. First, it allows the wearer's eyes to be more visible to someone who is looking at them. Without the coating, reflections are seen, similar to that experienced when viewing an eyeglass wearer on television and seeing the reflections of studio lights on the lenses. Second, the anti-reflective coating, by allowing more light to pass through a lens, also makes the vision through the lens more distinct. Without the coating, reflections are noticed around streetlights and headlights at night. The anti-reflective coating allows the lights to pass through without the glare or distortion.

In the computer-viewing environment, the anti-reflective coating will eliminate the glare and reflections in the eyeglass lenses that are caused by the surrounding lights. However, it will not affect the glare and reflections in the computer screen that are caused by the surrounding lights. This requires a screen anti-glare filter.

An anti-reflection coating, when applied to the eyeglass lenses of the computer user, allows for greater visual efficiency and greater visual comfort. With different qualities of anti-reflection coatings available, it is best for the computer user to consult with their eye care professional as to which design is best to use.

Contact Lenses

No presentation of visual correction for the computer user would be complete without a discussion of contact lenses. Contact lenses have become one of the prime methods of visual correction both inside and outside of the workplace. However, their use in the computer using environment brings with it special requirements and concerns.

Computer viewing, unlike reading documents, books, and magazines, requires the viewer to have a higher level of viewing angle. That is, the user's eyes must look higher in the field of view. Because of this difference, the eyes are open wider, creating more exposure of the eyes and greater evaporation of the tears. In addition, the user's blink rate is generally one third of the rate of the normal blink rate. This leads the computer user to have more frequent feelings of dry, irritated, and red eyes.

Erroneously, many wearers of contact lenses and their eye doctors conclude that contact lens wear is contraindicated in a computer-using environment. Nothing could be further from the truth. With the introduction of new contact lens materials and designs, wearers of contact lenses are now able to be fit with lenses that are resistant to dehydration, while maintaining clear, crisp vision.

Most often, contact lenses are fit for the wearer's distance correction requirements. However, as discussed previously, with increasing age individuals exhibit greater difficulty in near focusing. This need has been addressed by the contact lens industry with the introduction of the multifocal contact lenses. When fit and worn properly, they allow the wearer to see clearly at near, intermediate, and far distances.

Some contact lens wearers have been using a technique called "monovision," a term that describes a contact lens fit for distance vision on one eye and another for near vision on the other. While this sounds like a strange situation, it has proven to be a valuable technique for many contact lens wearers for many years. However, this technique does not take in the intermediate viewing distance of computer users.

Thus, it is only through a thorough discussion of the employee's needs, habits, and environment with an eye care professional that a decision can be made as to what lens design lens would be appropriate.

8

Vision in Industrial Settings

Bernard R. Blais

CONTENTS

Aspects of the Industrial Setting

The basic principles of industrial ophthalmology had been developed as far back as September 25, 1913 (Pizzarello, 1999; Resnick and Carris, 1924), when the National Safety Council was formed. The problem is that the basic principles, originally for the workplace, have not been thoroughly implemented in small businesses, nor in the home, on the streets, and in other public places, even though the National Committee for the Prevention of Blindness initiated a nationwide study in the latter part of 1923.

Pizzarello (1999), in his review, revealed that the early years of the twentieth century saw the emergence of an industrialized America. Injuries associated with this manufacturing environment were quite different from those sustained in the agrarian setting. It was in this context that the first attempts to prevent workplace injuries began. In New York State, eye injuries requiring more than one day's absence from work accounted for 15% of all industrial injuries; moreover, there was data that showed that 85% of injuries could be prevented with the adoption of appropriate protective eye wear (EEOC, 1992).

In 1924 Resnick et al. stated the following:

> The greatest influence for the elimination of the eye hazards of industrial occupations is, of course, the general industrial safety movement. There were undoubtedly, numerous plants where, because of several very costly eye accidents, greater attention was being given to the prevention of this particular type of accident than to the prevention of accidents in general. On the whole, however, the best results in the prevention of accidental injury to the eyes and in the conservation of vision through proper lighting and sanitation are to be found in those plants which are doing good all-round safety work. (Resnick and Carris, 1924)

In 1924 William Fellows Morgan, president of the National Committee for the Prevention of Blindness, organized in 1915, stated that from the beginning the Committee sought to bring the eye hazards of industrial occupations and the means of eliminating them to the attention of industry and of the country at large. The function of the National Committee for the Prevention of Blindness was not only in the industrial field, but in the general life of our country (Resnick and Carris, 1924).

In the early years of the twentieth century in England, Simeon Snell, M.D., began a systematic analysis of the needs of specialized workers (Snell, 1942). In the U.S., Albert Snell, M.D., pursued similar work. As industrialization reached its peak during the years of World War II, there emerged a parallel movement to improve eye safety with the introduction of the discipline of industrial ophthalmology.

The name associated with the pioneering work in this field is that of Hedwig Kuhn, M.D. Her work, *Industrial Ophthalmology* (Kuhn, 1946), was the state of the art in eye safety. Kuhn stressed the need to assess the vision needs of the worker and then match those needs to the ophthalmic evaluation conducted for that worker. Her research at Purdue University established standards that are still in use today. These analyses defined the specific vision needs of the worker, such as the stereo acuity of crane operators and the acuity needs of a fingerprint analyzer. She summarized the key elements of the process as

1. Selecting adequate pre-employment tests.
2. Providing periodic rechecks of specific groups.
3. Conducting a practical visual survey of the plant. (Kuhn, 1941)

At the same time, a major emphasis was placed on the development of a thorough eye protection program. The technology had changed little in the first 40 years of the century, and the biggest problem remained the issue of worker compliance.

Legal Attributes Related to Ocular Requirements

Today there are at least two legal requirements that employers must adhere to regarding visual requirements and safety.

1. The Rehabilitation Act of 1973 (Section 504 29 USC Para 794)/Americans with Disabilities Act of 1990 (ADA, 1990).
2. Occupational Health and Safety Acts of 1972 — The eye requirements of the law as incorporated in Sections 29CFR 1910.132 (OSHA, 1994) and 29CFR 1910.133, 1990.

The Prospective Worker

Each individual applying for a position in a large plant undergoes a complete physical appraisal. Part of this preplacement, post-offer survey is the ocular (vision) screening, which in the more progressive plants consists of a battery of tests supplied by a single screening or rating instrument. This is a far cry from the reading of a Snellen chart, badly illuminated, badly worn, badly distanced, and badly interpreted. The basic tests offered to the new employee consist of a series well-known to most of you, and of vital importance in industry as they help determine the worker's ability to meet the job's physical demands.

The results from these procedures are then, in a well-integrated program, matched against the visual requirements of the job. If the applicant fails to meet these, his visual skills are utilized in that occupation in which they will serve him and management in the best capacity. It is in this role that the eye care provider plays so keen a part, by interpreting from these tests the visual skills of the applicant. In large plants, the eye care provider interprets the findings of tests done by nontechnical personnel; in small organizations the provider performs the tests. In cooperation with the medical and personnel directors, the eye care provider uses the data to place the applicant in a job — actually fitting the eyes to the job.

In order to apply the preplacement examination findings, a detailed knowledge of the job is a must. Such information is derived from a visual analysis of the occupation.

These data, or visual skills demanded of the worker, are written into the job requirements and tabulated.

The practitioner must accomplish this visual survey in order to get into the shops, develop knowledge of the jobs, learn the shop language, and become familiar with the workers' daily environment. From this point on, the practitioner is of immeasurable aid to the medical director and the personnel director, who are trying to place a certain person in a certain job that will utilize the employee's skills to best advantage.

Prevention

General Principles

Harris (2003), in the American College of Occupational and Environmental Medicine Occupational Medicine Practice Guidelines, provides guidance on prevention.

Prevention of work-related health complaints should be a top priority for occupational health professionals. Workers presenting with work-related problems represent an opportunity to prevent recurrences in those workers (tertiary prevention), to mitigate the effects of current work-related hazards in order to reduce the duration of the problem (secondary prevention), and to prevent the same problems in co-workers and those in similar jobs (primary prevention). Different levels of certainty about the cause of the problem and differences in the severity of the adverse effects on health may justify different levels of response.

Work factors of the work environment suggest that worksite intervention to prevent recurrences and hasten recovery may well be appropriate. The occupational health practitioner should be aware, however, that many musculoskeletal, psychological, and other problems may be multi-factorial and are often caused by several work and nonwork-related factors in varying combinations. Many potentially work-related complaints result from work-related and personal factors. Some so-called personal factors are, in reality, a mismatch between the worker's abilities and job demands, or lack of *person–job fit*.

A cluster of cases in a work group suggests a greater probability of previously unidentified problems in work design or management. The practitioner's task in prevention is first to identify associated or causative workplace and personal factors. The practitioner should then suggest scientifically based selection and screening of personnel, personal protection, and task or job redesign, as well as treatment and disability management.

Preventive Strategies and Tactics

Different strategies are needed to provide a prevention program (Harris, 2003).

Primary Prevention

From a public health point of view, primary prevention is preferable to secondary and tertiary prevention. The primary prevention of work-related disorders depends on the reduction or elimination of exposure to factors causally associated with those disorders in individuals susceptible to such stressors.

The primary prevention of work-related complaints thus depends on reducing exposure to physical, personal, and psychosocial stressors. Primary preventive strategies based on maintaining activity and flexibility of vision, such as exercise breaks (or new vision activities from VDT) for workers performing assembly tasks, appear to be low cost and generally effective, based on physiologic principles. Strategies that improve work organization and management should also be addressed.

Work Design — Several general principles of work design are important to prevent musculoskeletal disorders and visual fatigue or injury. These include protection from hazards via engineering controls (effective barriers to hazards), use of personal protective equipment, administrative controls, and adjustment of workstations, tasks, and tools to the individual worker's size and work capacity.

Person–job fit is a basic principle that will markedly reduce occupational health concerns, the costs from lost productivity due to illness and injury, and medical costs. The same principles are used either to engineer jobs so that they fit many people or to adapt a job, task, or workstation to a specific person.

Jobs and workstations should be ergonomically designed so that they fit most workers' capacities. Workstations, equipment, or task components should be adjustable for workers of different stature, strength, and endurance to ensure a match between each worker and his or her tasks, thereby avoiding discomfort, loss of productivity, and injury. Management practices and psychosocial factors as they relate to person–job fit should also be assessed.

Workstations should be designed to avoid repetitive twisting of the neck to refer to written materials. This also helps prevent visual fatigue.

The personal protective equipment (PPE) should be designed to provide maximum visual ergonomics regardless of what position the employee is in.

Secondary Prevention

Secondary prevention is aimed at reducing disability and hastening recovery once a health concern has become apparent (Harris, 2003). This is a more targeted approach, in that it has become apparent which workers will develop complaints, illnesses, or injuries. Since secondary prevention involves working in partnership with the worker, the cornerstones of this process are two-way communication, addressing myths and misconceptions, managing expectations, bilateral or trilateral planning, and managing the episode and the situation. Modified or limited duty is important to return workers to the worksite and prevent social isolation and de-conditioning.

Tertiary Prevention

Tertiary prevention in the work setting involves preventing recurrences in a patient who has had a previous episode (Harris, 2003). The first action should be to evaluate the job or tasks and the person–job fit and then modify the job, tasks, or workstation as necessary. Repetitions, abnormal postures (especially the corrective lens type in workers with presbyopia), and other ergonomic problems should be addressed. If the individual cannot do the job as originally designed due to an impairment, then reasonable accommodation should be attempted. If that is not possible, job placement elsewhere or retraining may be indicated.

Beyond Prevention: Promotion

Keeney (2002), in his *Duane's Clinical Ophthalmology* chapter, "The Eye and the Workplace: Special Considerations," reflects the need for promotion.

In the United States in the early 1980s, there was marked intensification in the field of preventive ophthalmology, both as an academic discipline and as an institutional commitment. With this has come a governmental and industrial emphasis on health promotion, including on-the-job or worksite health promotion. Major industries are fostering this in an effort to contain medical program costs. To be successful, these programs must be voluntary and stem from a positive commitment through all levels of management, employees and unions (Grundy, 1981; Kuhn, 1944; Brownell, 1947).

An initial period of data gathering is necessary to identify medical, health, and ophthalmic problems particular to a given industry or plant. This investigation includes not only risks of specific trauma to the eyes, but also surveys to determine what kinds of promotions are of interest to and desired by the employees. It is often done as an extension of pre-existing medical screening, injury prevention, and on-the-job initial medical care. Such an approach emphasizes what is already going on in a positive way and may identify untapped resources of people, materials, and equipment within a company or a plant.

The programs require that a qualified and enthusiastic person be given clear responsibility for developing promotional activities that integrate with the specific activities of the plant. Management should participate in the activities as well as sanction the program. Some clear and realistic measurable goals should be established and the program given an initial trial period of at least three years. All aspects of the program should be voluntary but should have the official support of public relations officers and communications departments within the industry. Some aspects of the program should be offered on company time, and management should decide whether or not it is to be presented as part of an ongoing employee benefit package or as a separate undertaking.

A Basic Industrial Visual Program

The Joint Industrial Ophthalmology Committee in June 1944, as reported (*Duane's Clinical Ophthalmology* 2002), outlined a basic industrial visual program, which is essentially still used in the twenty-first century as a guide for eye practitioners who may be interested in the industrial field.

Essentials of Visual Functions

In 1944, Kuhn reported in her textbook that (occupational) industrial ophthalmology, as a special field, had not been previously dealt with as a comprehensive treatis (Kuhn, 1944). She attempted to address much of the essential information relating to the various problems that confront industry and that also bear a special relationship to ophthalmology. In 1942, Dr. Albert Snell stated: "Good vision is that degree of visual function ability which is adequate to perform the task presented" (Snell, 1942).

Kuhn (1944) recommended a research project. What facts about eyes were important? When obtained, how were these facts to be interpreted? When interpreted, how could they best be used in rehabilitation efforts? How could they be used in an effort to step up production? How could they be harnessed to reduce accidents? (Pizzarello, 1999; Snell, 1942)

As far back as 1945, Kuhn stated:

> An essential and as yet hardly touched part of an intelligent appraisal of industrial eye problems (and actually that part on which all other steps of a program are based), was a detailed visual job analysis. To know what a given pair of eyes must be able to do in order to place new employees according to their visual skills; in order to correct any defect properly for that work (if refractive correction is indicated); in order to choose the right type of protective equipment, one must see each and every job and codify its essential characteristics. (Kuhn, 1946)

We had to wait until 1990, however, when the Americans with Disabilities Act was enacted, to legally implement this analysis, yet no current published document provides such analyses for all occupations.

Kuhn (1944) also stated that in establishing a testing procedure industry, three main objectives were required: selecting adequate pre-employment tests; providing periodic rechecks of special groups; and conducting a practical visual survey of the plant.

In this broad discussion of an eye program for industry, the author seeks to open one more door that had been unfamiliar to the eye care professional. Information about a worker's visual skills, such as acuity, muscle balance, and visual performance at near-point distances, is of first importance to management as well as to the medical department. The constant and terrific effort for capacity-plus production, for speedy production, for the elimination of the scrap heaps of spoiled material, is often based squarely on these visual skills.

By and large, neither industry nor the eye care professional is properly informed on what actually constitutes a proper eye protection plan, especially small industry, and for this reason a rather complete discussion of an eye qualification and protection program is included. In the 1940s industrial eye programs that included such questions as: What is proper illumination? What are a few of the high spots of the medico-legal angles in the handling of eye cases? What are the problems of radiation, and "flashes?" Resnick's 1924 statement is still true today: "There are still countless plants, whose operations present serious eye hazards, in which no goggles are available even for the workman who, on his own initiative, might apply for them. There are many plants where workmen wear goggles on their caps or in their pockets except when 'the boss is watching them.'" (Resnick and Carris,

1924) How can we renew the emphasis placed by Resnick and others in today's eye safety and conservation program?

Performing Essential Functions With or Without Accommodation

The Americans with Disabilities Act of 1990 (ADA, 1990), as implemented in most facilities in July of 1992 under Title 1 on employability, requires that the individual must be able to perform the essential functions of the position with or without accommodation without significant risk or direct threat to themselves and to others. In presentations to AAO and the American Occupational Health Conference, Blais discussed the relevance of visual requirements to efficiency and safety. These workplace requirements are no different from what would be expected and desired from one planning to drive a car, play sports, practice hobbies, or perform hazardous duties at school or on the farm.

The Requirements of the Rehabilitation Act

The federal law most relevant to decisions regarding the vision standards for applicants is the Rehabilitation Act of 1973. The other federal law relevant to decisions is the Americans with Disabilities Act.

The Rehabilitation Act of 1973 prohibits discrimination against people with handicaps by employers who receive federal financial assistance. The Americans with Disabilities Act was modeled after the Rehabilitation Act of 1973. Essentially, it extends the provisions against discrimination to private employers. It prohibits discrimination against people with disabilities by private employers whether or not they receive federal financial assistance. The Americans with Disabilities Act also is more explicit and detailed about what employers must do to include people with disabilities in their workforce and what is meant by reasonable accommodations (ADA, 1990).

The Rehabilitation Act makes it unlawful for an employer that receives federal financial assistance to exclude, or otherwise discriminate against, persons solely because of a handicap. The presence of a handicapping condition is not a permissible ground for assuming a person is unable to function effectively in a particular job. Handicapped persons who meet all the employment criteria except for the challenged discriminatory criterion and who can perform the essential functions of the job with or without reasonable accommodations cannot be rejected from a job simply because of a handicap.

The determination of whether an individual with a disability is qualified to perform a particular job is to be made at the time of the employment decision. This determination should be based on the capabilities of the individual with a disability at the time of the employment decision, and should not be based on speculation that the employee may become unable to perform the job in the future or may cause increased health insurance premiums or workers' compensation costs. See the Department of Justice and Equal

Employment Opportunity Commission (EEOC)'s *Americans With Disabilities Handbook,* Interpretive Guidance, Section 1630.2(m) (EEOC, 1992).

Essential Functions of the Job

The "essential functions" of a particular job may be determined by using the job description developed by the employer or by relying on those familiar with the particular job. Not all job functions articulated by an employer are essential functions, nor are all employer qualifications to be accepted as essential.

While legitimate physical qualifications may be essential to the performance of certain jobs, that determination and the determination of whether or not accommodation is possible to overcome any physical limitations must be made by scrutinizing the evidence carefully.

Reasonable Accommodation

If a handicapped person is unable to meet the employer's requirements, it is the employer's obligation to investigate and determine whether a reasonable accommodation can be made to enable the person to perform the job. Reasonable accommodations may include but are not limited to acquisition or modifications of equipment or devices, and appropriate adjustment or modifications of examinations, training materials, or policies. If reasonable accommodations do exist, these should be used rather than excluding the handicapped person. A reasonable accommodation may require an employer to accept minor inconvenience or to bear more than an insignificant economic cost in making allowance for an applicant's handicap.

An employer may require, as a qualification standard, that an individual not pose a significant risk or direct threat to the health or safety of himself/ herself or others. The determination that an individual with a disability poses a direct threat should be made on an individual case-by-case basis. The determination may also be based on a reasonable medical judgment that relies on the most current medical knowledge and on the best available objective evidence. In determining whether an individual would pose a direct threat, the factors to be considered include the duration of the risk, the nature and severity of the potential harm, and the likelihood that the potential harm will occur.

The law requires that consideration must rely on objective factual evidence — not on subjective perceptions, irrational fears, patronizing attitudes, or stereotypes — about the nature or effect of a particular disability, or of disability generally.

If an individual poses a direct threat as a result of a disability, the employer must determine whether a reasonable accommodation would either eliminate the risk or reduce it to an acceptable level. An employer is not permitted to deny employment to an individual with a disability merely because of a slightly increased risk. The risk can only be considered when it poses a significant risk. A significant risk is a risk that has a high probability of substantial harm.

Burden of Proof — Preponderance of the Evidence

Before an employer can exclude an individual with a handicap, the employer must meet its burden of demonstrating by a preponderance of the evidence* that the handicapped individual cannot perform a job with or without reasonable accommodations. Handicapped people should be eligible for employment unless they cannot perform the job with or without reasonable accommodation.

The visual requirements for a given position have been the subject of discussion as far back as 1945 when a Committee on Industrial Ophthalmology of the American Academy of Ophthalmology and Otolaryngology (AAOO) chaired by Dr. Hedwig Kuhn published a series of articles on industrial eye problems in consecutive issues of the *Transactions of Ophthalmology and Otolaryngology* (TAAOO, 1941; 1942a; 1942b; 1943; 1944). Drs. Tiffin and Wirt, in their study, now considered the Purdue University Study, analyzed the relationship of accident-free performance and stated there must be some minimum requirements or standards of performance on the visual examination which may be demanded of any employee who is assigned to such jobs.

Dr. Stump (1946) reviewed the employee's visual performance and compared with visual standards. He found that the percentage increase in accidents by extreme deviation from the standard was 106%, 43% for moderate deviation, and 31% for negligible deviation from the standard. Because we are now raising the question of "good vision," we are talking about a function which, in the majority of the cases, can be improved by professional attention. Dr. Albert Snell (1942) stated: "*Good vision is that degree of visual function ability which is adequate to perform the visual task presented.*" Evidence is now available to show that visual functions are important factors in safety. Thus, bringing individuals up to satisfactory visual standards, will reduce accidents. Kuhn (1946), Tiffin and Wirt (1945), Stump (1946), and others have studied visual skills in relation to job performance in many types of work, and the results have indicated that visual skills of one sort or another are

---

* What does a "preponderance of evidence" mean? To establish a fact by a preponderance of the evidence means to prove that the fact is more likely true than not true. A preponderance of the evidence means the greater weight of the evidence. It refers to the quality and persuasiveness of the evidence, not to the number of witnesses or documents. So long as the scales tip, however slightly, in favor of the party with this burden of proof — that what the party claims is more likely true than not true — then it will have been proved by a preponderance of evidence. Department of Justice and EEOC's *Americans With Disabilities Act Handbook*, Interpretive Guidance, Section 1630.2(r); Strathie v. Department of Transportation, 716 F.2d 227 (3rd Cir. 1983); N.Y.A.R.C. v. Carey, 612 F.2d 644, 649 (2d Cir. 1979); Modern Federal Jury Instructions, Vol. 3, ¶73.01, Instruction 73.2.

probably one of the most universal and frequent factors affecting job performance, and job performance can often be predicted, to some extent, on the basis of the visual skills.

Elements of Ocular Function

Ocular function is important to the safety, health, and efficiency of industry workers. The Joint Industrial Ophthalmology Committee of AAOO (1944) set forth the following elements of visual function (now called ocular function requirements):

Basic elements of visual function include information needed for industrial employees' records. It is important that records be kept of these findings when using any battery of binocular tests because this enables industry to note changes.

1. Acuity

   Monocular and binocular

   Distance and near*

   With and without correction

2. Stereopsis — Techniques for testing stereopsis in a binocular instrument have been greatly improved.

3. Color Perception — Color perception is important in many industries. One should know what color deficiencies interfere with safety and efficiency.**

4. Muscle Balance — (distance and near). The common term "muscle balance" is chosen for the sake of presenting the concept of binocular balance to the layman. The examination of muscle function should be for vertical and horizontal phorias.

   a. General limits of normal functional balance should be set for far and for near.

   b. Determination of what is adequate from a comfort, efficiency, and safety viewpoint for any one individual should be determined by the nature of the occupation. No absolutes are possible but the degree of interference with comfort is an index, and this must be used in judging whether the defect is a minor one or one that needs correction for industrial employment.

---

* Near vision is considered at this time as 16 in. and intermediate vision is considered at this time as intermediate distance between 20 ft and 16 in. where an individual performs specific tasks.

** The universal testing for red and green must be supplemented with blue and yellow for many tasks. Visual screeners generally test for only red and green.

Visual Screening, as defined by a conjoint proposal from the American Academy of Pediatrics, the American Academy of Ophthalmology, the Eye and Vision Committee of the American College of Occupational and Environmental Medicine, and the American Academy of Pediatric Ophthalmology and Strabismology (1998), is as follows:

- The key element is determination of screening visual acuity, both quantitative and bilateral.
- This service must employ graduated visual acuity stimuli that allow quantitative determination of visual acuity (e.g., Snellen Chart).
- It may include screening determination of contrasts sensitivity, ocular alignment, color vision, and visual fields.

Current Procedure Terminology Codes for Visual Screening

In the American Medical Association Current Procedure Terminology (AMA CPT) code guidelines for visual screening (E/M Preventive Medicine Codes) effective March 1998, the AMA has designated Preventive Medicine CPT Codes for Visual Screening.

Prior to the determination of AMA CPT codes, none were available to family physicians, pediatricians, occupational health physicians, ophthalmologists, or optometrists for vision screening reimbursements. In March 1998, the AMA Department of Coding and Nomenclature recommended the use of preventive medicine CPT codes along with evaluation and management codes to report this service (personal communication, March 4, 1998).

This battery of tests should be regarded as screening tests, to detect substandard visual qualifications. They are not diagnostic! Follow-up procedures that are necessary may be briefly outlined as (TAAOO, 1944):

1. Employees who, on screening tests, have a high standard of performance for the specific job can be so certified to the proper placement personnel.
2. Employees who appear to have limitations of visual skills that are likely to affect their work should be referred to a competent professional who has knowledge of the visual requirements of the various job classifications in the plant, or who is specifically informed as to the type of job for which the employee is being considered or presently holds.

Current Ocular (Visual) Screening Testing Method

The majority of the visual tests required may be provided by use of visual screeners. Currently, the following instruments are available:

Titmus Model 2a Screener (Titmus Optical, Inc., Petersburg, VA):

- VA. D, INT. (20 to 40 in.) near: monocular and binocular
- Color vision red or green
- Muscle balance — heterophoria or heterotropia, horizontal and vertical
- Stereopsis
- Peripheral vision — horizontal plane

Stereo Optical Model Optec 5500 or remote control Optic 5500P Vision Tests (Stereo Optical Co., Inc., Chicago, IL):

- VA. D, INT. (20-36 in.) near: monocular and binocular
- Color vision red or green
- Muscle balance — heterophoria or heterotropia, horizontal and vertical
- Stereopsis
- Peripheral vision — horizontal plane
- Contrast sensitivity available

The Department of Defense utilizes an Armed Forces Visual Screener — Bausch & Lomb Ortho-Rater, Stereo Optical Company (Chicago, IL) Model Optec 2300 Armed Forces Vision Tester. Other instruments currently in use but not being manufactured at the present time include Bausch & Lomb, American Optical instruments previously described. The tests may be provided through individual separate instruments.

A software-based program, "The Eye-CEE System for Computer Users" is a product of the Department of Optometry and Visual Science at City University in London. It combines an on-screen questionnaire with a series of visual tests to determine whether a computer user is having visual stress at the workstation. It carries out a comprehensive analysis of the user's visual performance under normal viewing conditions. It is available in the U.S. from Corporate Vision Consulting (Encinitas, CA).

General Visual Standards

Tiffin (1947), in his textbook *Industrial Psychology*, stated that the visual requirements for a given position have been the subject of discussion since 1945, when the Joint Committee on Industrial Ophthalmology of the AAOO stated that there must be some minimum requirements or standards of performance on the visual examination that may be demanded of any employee. Dr. Kuhn stated that the concept of differentiating between the separate visual standards and relating each to the requirement of a given job, can be vividly illustrated. These visual requirements for employment on certain jobs or in certain plants may be set in one of two ways:

- Observations — set by someone's opinion as to what test is to be used and what degree of performance on this test is to be required for specific jobs, based on more or less (and sometimes not on any) direct and expert observation of the job in question.

- Statistical — A set of statistical facts that determine which tests and what minimum levels of performance on these tests will most adequately identify the worker who will be potentially better on the job in question.

The problem of setting visual standards on a factual or statistical basis is essentially one of establishing individual differences in job performance and individual differences in visual skills, and determining how these differences in job performance are dependent on differences in visual skills, and how they may be predicted, to some extent, on the basis of the visual skill test. Questions to be answered are:

1. What vision tests are related to specific measures of performance on a specific job and are the results reproducible?
2. What degree of performance on these tests is requisite for average performance on a job, and what degree is desirable for maximum performance?
3. What difference in average job performance for the group as a whole could be expected if all workers on the job had the requisite or desirable visual skills?

Visual Requirements of Jobs

Tiffin (1943), in *Industrial Psychology*, stated that it is apparent from casual observation that jobs differ in the visual demands they make upon the worker. These variations are both qualitative and quantitative. Consider the job of crane operator where the worker is required to see clearly at a distance of perhaps 60 to 100 ft ahead in order accurately to set down a load in a narrowly prescribed area. Compare this job in respect to visual demands with that of a radio assembler who is required to see clearly materials very close to his eyes in order to be able to quickly fit together the intricate system of small parts and wires that go into a radio. The job of crane operator makes severe demands upon the worker's ability to see detail at a great distance. The ability to differentiate such detail close up is much less important to the job. The radio assembler, on the other hand, finds these two types of visual demands reversed. He is required to differentiate minute detail at close range and has relatively much less need for such visual ability at a greater distance.

In the same manner as the demands for acuity at different distances vary from the job of crane operator to the job of radio assembler, so the demands for other visual skills vary from one job to another. Some jobs require relatively high degrees of proficiency in certain types of visual skills combined with lesser requirements for proficiency in other visual skills. Thus, we have a qualitative difference between jobs with respect to the types of visual skill required in their performance.

Just as jobs vary in the types of visual skill they require, they also vary in the degree of any one visual skill that may be required.

The adequate use of a battery of visual skills tests in the selection and placement of industrial workers requires an accurate method of determining both the type and quantity of visual skills demanded by various industrial jobs. The visual requirements for different jobs cannot be established adequately by mere observation of the job activity. They can, however, be established by the methods of test validation.

Observation Technique

Visual Task Analysis

Analysis of the visual factors required for the task is of crucial importance and ideally any analysis should be carried out at the place of work, e.g., factory or office. From the subsequent analysis, the important visual factors can be identified. This fulfills the requirement of ADA 90 and OSHA 29CFR 1910.132.

Koven reports (1947–1948) that the job analysis for visual requirements entails a careful survey of each component part of a given job in relation to the employee's visual skills involved in the performance of that job. This type of analysis requires a broad knowledge of visual abilities and limitations (problems of accommodation, convergence, presbyopia, coordination, muscle balance, etc.), lighting, physical factors, and the host of eye hazards of the particular operation. This type of survey is best done as a cooperative undertaking in which the plant medical director, the consulting eye physician, production, illuminating, and safety engineers, the personnel director, and supervisors make their respective contributions as necessary. In some instances, one person with unusual knowledge and experience can qualify for these various skills. The information included in job analysis for visual requirements may vary somewhat, but in general the following points are covered in Table 8.1.

TABLE 8.1

Checklist of Visual Job Analysis

1. Job description (including qualifications relative to type of training and skills) with standard code number.
2. Distance or distances (distance for acuity and/or near acuity) in inches or feet from eyes of worker to point of operation, fixed or changing.
3. Motion of work (distance and near muscle balance): slow or rapid rotation, vertical or horizontal, fixed or intermittent.
4. Size of central working area, depth perception factors (stereopsis).
5. Type of visual attention required: fixed or changing, casual or concentrated, detailed or gross (or listed as perfect, average or defective permissible; or as class A, B, or C).
6. Colors to be perceived and discriminated.
7. Foot candles of illumination at workpoint, as well as in surrounding area. Direction of light (note any harmful shadows). Reflected or direct glares (to be eliminated if possible). Brightness ratios (avoid sharp contrasts).
8. Color of light source and work area (functional painting, etc.).
9. Type of working surface: glossy or non-glossy, slightly or grossly uneven. Angle of working surface. Position of work in relation to normal level of eyes, viz., does worker have to look down, ahead, or upward (determine whether bifocals are permissible or a handicap).
10. Eye hazards: flying objects, particles of dusts, fumes, splashing chemicals, or molten metal; airborne matter; radiation, etc.
11. Type of eye protection required.

Visual Ergonomics of the Workplace*

Studies indicate that the visual complaints occur in 50 to 90% of workers who use VDTs. The vision problems result from visual inefficiencies and in eye-related symptoms the causes of which are a combination of the individual visual problems and poor visual ergonomics. The problems occur whenever the visual demands of the task exceed the visual abilities of the individual. The problems are very real, very prevalent, and we know the basis for most of the problems. The visual symptoms can be resolved for the most part with good visual ergonomics through the management of the environment and by providing proper visual care to the computer worker. Ergonomics is the science of designing the workplace, machines and work tasks with the capabilities and limitations of the human being in mind (see Figure 8.1).

North (1993) states that the ability to perform most tasks depends on many visual and nonvisual variables, and the factors that influence the visual performance can be listed as follows: the visual capability of the individual, the visibility of the task, the psychological and general physiological factors.

---

* Koven, A.L., The Right Eyes for the Right Job, TAAOO, September/October 1947, V. 52, 1947–1948, p. 46-50.

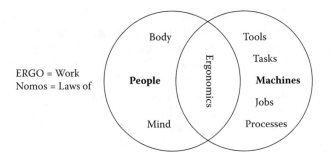

FIGURE 8.1

Ergonomics — Science of designing the workplace machines and work tasks with capabilities and limitations of the human being in mind.

It is not within the scope of this chapter to deal with the third group of factors in depth, although psychological and general physiological factors, such as motivation, intelligence, general health, etc., should not be forgotten, because they can all influence the visual performance. This chapter deals with the first two variables — visual capabilities and the visibility of the task. The visual capabilities have already been discussed.

Visibility of Tasks

North (1993) noted that the ability to perform a task safely, efficiently, and comfortably depends upon its visibility, as well as on the visual capabilities of the employee, as outlined earlier. Naturally, the better the visibility, the easier it is to perform the task, and the factors that influence the visibility of a task can be listed as follows:

- Size of task
- Distance of task
- Illumination
- Glare
- Contrast
- Color
- Time available to view task
- Movement of the task
- Atmospheric conditions

Static Acuity

Static visual acuity is the capacity for seeing distinctly the details of a stationary object. This should be related directly to size and distance of the small detail required to be seen in the assigned task.

The time available to view the letters, etc., will influence the visual acuity measured. It has been estimated that a person can transmit up to 10 bits/sec (a bit is a unit of information) of visually displayed information. This is a very small amount of information, when it is estimated that the human sensory system has a capacity to transmit millions of bits/sec. Therefore, it is not the input of the visual system that limits the visual performance but the processing, decision-making, and motor output. Letters can usually be recognized in less than a second and, obviously, the better the illumination and the larger the letter, the faster the recognition time.

Verneir Acuity

The type of visual acuity discussed so far has been form acuity, the ability to discriminate between two small parts of an object. However, in some occupations line detail is required, for example, the use of micrometers or precision gauges requires the discrimination of a break in contour or alignment, i.e., vernier acuity. The visual system is extremely sensitive to these details and it is approximately one twentieth of the corresponding angle for details to be resolved in form acuity (Grundy, 1988). If the form acuity for a certain distance is known, then it is relatively easy to calculate the equivalent visual angle for vernier acuity and the actual size that may be resolved, and vice versa. Misalignments of segments of a divided line of approximately three seconds of arc can be detected at moderately high levels of illumination, whereas the minimum angle of resolution is from 30 to 60 seconds of arc (Westheimer, 1987).

There are numerous factors, according to North (1993) — physical, physiological, and psychological — that can influence the ability of the visual system to see details. These can be listed as follows: luminance, contrast, spectral nature of light, size and intensity of surrounding field, region of retina stimulated, distance and size of object, time available to see object, glare foggy/steamy atmosphere, refractive error, pupil size, age, attention, IQ, boredom, ability to interpret blurred images, general health, and emotional state (Riggs, 1965; Westheimer, 1987). Some of the major factors will now be discussed.

Size of Task

The size of the critical detail of the task (Boyce and Simons, 1977) needs to be taken into account so that the angle subtended at the eye, and hence the visual acuity necessary to perform the task comfortably and efficiently can be calculated. The retinal image size of any object is inversely proportional to its distance from the eye. Therefore, objects may differ greatly in physical dimensions but form similar retinal image size due to the fact that they are viewed at different distances (see Figure 8.2). So, while the visual acuity may be the same, the demands made upon accommodation and convergence may

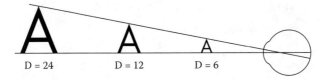

FIGURE 8.2
Relationship of size and distance from eye-retinal image size of object A is inversely proportional to its distance from the eye.

be different. A very small object may have to be placed very close for the detail to be large enough to be resolved, but this will require good accommodation and convergence.

Distance of the Task

Naturally, the distance of the task (Boyce and Simons, 1977) from the observer and the size of the detail of the task affect the retinal image size, and hence the visual acuity required to distinguish it. The distance of the task also determines the level of accommodation and convergence and the degree of uncorrected refractive error or phoria that may be tolerated. Working distances may be classified as: far (>2 m), intermediate-to-near (<2 m and >30 cm), and very near (<30 cm) (Grundy, 1988). Examples of tasks involving far working distances include driving a vehicle and flying an airplane; intermediate-to-near tasks include secretarial work, VDT operating, and lathe operating; and very near tasks include sewing, micro-electronics assembly work, and watch repairing (see Figure 8.3).

The amount of accommodation decreases with age, and generally, after their mid-40s workers require a spectacle prescription to focus near objects clearly and comfortably. As the range of accommodation reduces with age, the range of clear vision through the various near vision powers becomes smaller.

It is worthwhile mentioning that workers with poor visual acuity may also benefit from increased lighting levels (Silver et al., 1980; Julian, 1984) and from more magnification to increase the retinal image size.

Illumination

Proper illumination is important and it should be evaluated for each task. The relationship between illumination on the task and performance achieved will vary according to the type of task (Boyce and Simons, 1977). In summary, the effect of illumination upon task performance will vary according to:

- The visual details of the task
- The extent to which the visual part of the task determines the overall performance.

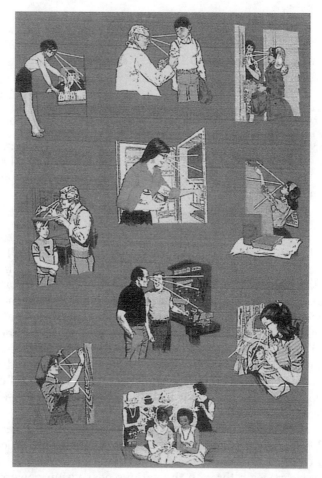

FIGURE 8.3
Potential Visual Task. Distance that requires good accommodation and convergence. (Courtesy of Essilor of America.)

The greater the visual difficulty, the greater the effect of the illuminance. Whereas in a task such as audio typing, where there is only a small visual component, the effect of illuminance upon the overall task performance will be small. The effect of illuminance is dependent on the needs of the task, reflectance of surfaces in the area, and, to some extent, the age of the worker. Older workers generally require brighter lighting for visual discrimination. In general, illuminance of 70 to 80 foot candles (ft-c) is needed for general office work, 100-150 ft-c for visually intensive tasks, and up to 500 to 1000 ft-c for very fine tasks (Boyce and Simons, 1977).

Glare

The effect of veiling reflections and the complexity of the task have a significant effect on job performance (Boyce and Simons, 1977) Veiling reflections are due to light from a high luminance surface, such as a luminaire, being reflected from a specular surface, which is being viewed. These veiling reflections cause a reduction in performance due to the decreased contrast created on the task by the superimposed reflections.

Lighting geometry should be configured to avoid glare. Glare on VDT screens, for example, should be reduced by:

- Placing visual display terminals out of direct line with or facing windows
- Using window films and coverings
- Using dull, textured surfaces
- Reducing ambient lighting to below 500 lux (18-46 ft-c) and using supplemental lighting where needed
- Using indirect lighting
- Using parabolic louvers on fluorescent lights
- Shielding auxiliary lighting
- Using eye shades

Visual discomfort from glare and other sources accumulates during the workday, so task rotation may be a reasonable preventive measure if other measures are not possible or reasonable. Glare is a known problem in presbyopic individuals where early cataract changes in the lens may have developed.

Contrast

The eye detects objects by responding to the differing levels of illumination at the target edges, or contrast (Boyce and Simons, 1977):

$$\text{contrast} = \frac{\text{background illumination} - \text{target illumination}}{\text{background illumination}}$$

To determine the optimum illumination levels for a task, the contrast and size need to be measured and, as mentioned, it is not easy to measure the contrast of a practical task. These recommendations apply to tasks of normal contrast and reflectance. If, however, the contrast or reflectances are low, or if mistakes made due to wrong perception are likely to be dangerous or costly, the recommended illumination should be increased. Refractive surgery (i.e., LASIK, for example) frequently has postoperative complications of decreased contrast sensitivity and increased glare. The glare predominately at night is also seen in bright sunlight.

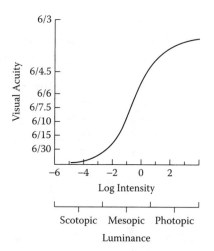

FIGURE 8.4
Luminence and contrast – The relationship between visual acuity and luminance (measured in millilamberts). (Koneg's data reported by Heck 1934.) (From North RV. Work and the Eye. Oxford, England, Oxford University Press, 1993. With permission.)

Studies by Blackwell and Blackwell (1971) concerning the visibility of tasks have influenced the American codes for lighting. The initial experiments investigated the threshold detection of static disc targets, and later experiments involved the detection of dynamic targets. The dynamically presented targets were believed to create conditions more similar to a practical task. More recent studies have investigated the effects of lighting upon the visual performance of a 20- to 30-year-old age group (Blackwell and Blackwell 1980). Older individuals require more light than younger ones to perform a similar task (Boyce and Simons, 1977).

Luminance and Contrast

Two major factors that influence visual acuity are luminance and contrast. The influence of luminance upon visual acuity is shown in Figure 8.4. The capacity of the visual system to resolve details increases with increasing luminance, although there is a level beyond which visual acuity does not increase; in fact, it may diminish due to disability glare. Contrast has a maximal effect on visual acuity at low levels of illumination but a minimal effect at high levels.

Spotten, Hutchings, and Hartel, in their guidelines of ophthalmology, state that the graph of visual acuity plotted against contrast shows the rapid improvement in acuity as contrast increases and the difference that background illumination makes to the acuity under the same conditions of contrast. In Figure 8.5, the upper curve is plotted at a higher background illumination than the lower curve. As contrast increases, the two merge and the illumination difference becomes irrelevant. Marked above the curves are

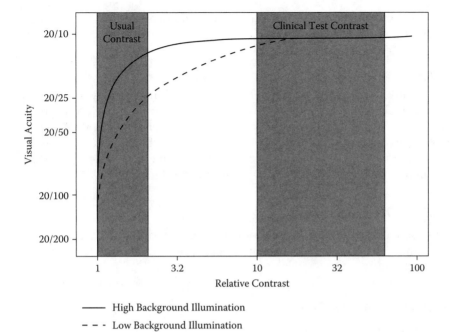

FIGURE 8.5

Visual acuity versus contrast shows rapid improvement in acuity as contrast increases. The upper curve is plotted at a higher background illumination than the lower curve. As contrast increases the two merge and the illumination difference becomes irrelevant. Marked above the curves are the contrast ranges of clinical test material and normal printed materials such as newsprint. From this, one can see the patients see clearer under test conditions using high-contrast typeface than they do at home, where ambient lighting may also be reduced. (Reprinted from Spalton DJ, Hitchings, RA, Hunter, PA. *Slide Atlas of Ophthalmology.* Copyright 1984, with permission from Elsevier.)

the contrast ranges of clinical test material and normal printed materials such as newsprint. From this, one can see that patients may see more clearly under test conditions using high-contrast typeface than they do at home, where ambient lighting may also be reduced. In clinical acuity tests, black letters are displayed on a white background giving a contrast value of approximately 80 to 85%. In the normal eye under photopic conditions, the threshold contrast is about 1%. In essence, clinics testing patients with old beaten up, yellowish visual acuity charts and very poor illumination (less than 7p.c.) are not recording the true visual acuity but instead 3 or 4 times below true visual acuity performed under more standard procedures.

The following example relates the association of distance and decreased contrast. The eye with a visual acuity of 20/40 visualizes a 1.0 mm target at 14 in. (35 cm). At 28 in., doubling the distance without change in size will require a visual acuity of 20/20 with high contrast using Figure 8.2. Working at moderate contrasts would require a visual acuity of 20/05. This visual acuity is not readily available in most human beings. In essence, doubling the distance doubles the visual requirement and decreasing the contrast also doubles the visual requirement.

Color

The ability to discriminate colors is particularly influenced by age and illumination. It has been shown that with age there are more errors in hue discrimination in the blue-green and red regions (Verriest et al. 1962). Similar effects have been found by Boyce (1977), who also found that the older age group made more errors in sorting the hues in the FM 100 hue test and that the number of errors decreased with increasing illumination.

Atmospheric Conditions

Atmospheric conditions in such industries as foundries and mining, where there may be dust, smoke, or steam will reduce visibility due to the absorption of light.

Steps in Setting Standard

Observations Techniques

After analysis of the visual task allowing the important visual factors to be determined, a standard can be set by either: (1) choosing a standard believed to be necessary to work efficiently and safely, e.g., Visual Acuity 6/12 (20/40), distinguish principal colors, which can be tested by relating visual competence to job competence as described previously; or (2) insisting on the normal level of visual capabilities for each factor chosen, e.g., Visual Acuity 6/6 (20/20), normal color vision. This approach would exclude some who were capable of performing the task comfortably.

Statistical Methods

Joseph Tiffin and his associates in the Division of Education and Applied Psychology, Purdue University, approached the problem of determining visual standards on a statistical basis. This involved testing a number of employees on a job — employees of all degrees of ability and achievement. These employees are classified on the basis of production, quality, rating, or whatever measures of job success are available, into categories from "definitely superior" to "definitely inferior." Then the visual characteristics of the different groups are compared in order to determine what visual skills the superior workers possess that inferior workers do not possess, or possess to a lesser degree. Since measurements of job performance are influenced by the amount of training and experience on the job, as well as by aptitudes and skills, careful handling of the data is needed to surmount these and other factors.

Visual Factors for Specific Tasks

North (1993) states there are occasions when on-site analysis is not possible. A logical method for determining the visual factors required for a particular task has been proposed by Grundy (1987) and is designed to act as a simple reference guide for use by optometrists in a consulting room (North, 1993; Table 2.1).

From the knowledge of the distance and size of the critical detail of the task, the visual acuity necessary to discriminate the smallest detail can be determined. This can be calculated easily from a simple graphical method using a nomogram, shown in Figure 8.6. For example, a task has a critical detail of 0.6 mm and it is viewed at 70 cm. When a straight line is drawn through these values it will intercept the right-hand scale to indicate that the corresponding visual angle is 3.0 min of arc and the minimum visual acuity required is 6/18 (20/60). It is important to remember that the values given are a measure of the resolving power of the eye and higher standards are required for the task to be carried out for prolonged periods of time. It has been suggested that the visual acuity necessary for a demanding task should be approximately twice the minimum value (Grundy, 1981). Therefore, in the above case, a visual acuity of 6/9 (20/30) is advised. Some authorities have advised a three-times size enlargement for comfortable viewing. The employee can often move closer to the task, increasing the angular size to the eye, but this depends on the amount of accommodation and convergence available. The older presbyopic employee, who has a reduced amount of accommodation, may need an intermediate and a near prescription, depending on the distance of the task. If an employee is diagnosed with "low" or subnormal vision, enlargement of the task is even more critical. This condition must be dealt with on a case-by-case basis.

Statistical Techniques

General

What we are actually dealing with in all screening tests, in job evaluation, and in the study of the individual elements of seeing considered as skills, is studying and judging *visual performance*. Substandard performance is not a substitute term for a clinical defect.

The statisticians have shown that by careful study of the visual skills found to be associated with successful employees on the payrolls, one can secure data so that one can predict the future success of comparable applicants. Generally speaking, that is the actual basis from which pre-employment standards are built. Medical people are trained on the whole to deal with sick, handicapped, and physically unsuccessful people. Their approach to examinations of a physical organ, such as the eye, and its relationship to a given task, is to think of the defects that prevent a person from performing

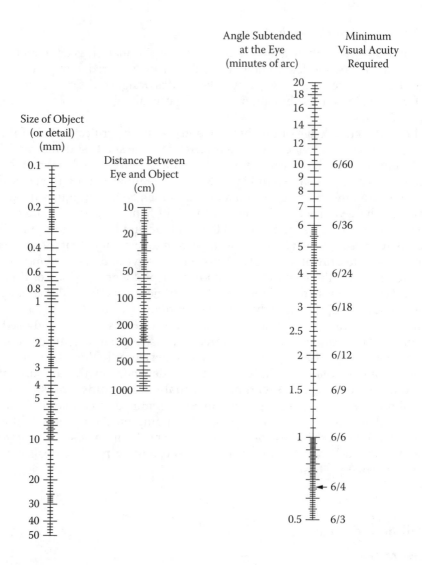

FIGURE 8.6
Nomogram for finding the visual angle subtended by objects of which the size and distance vary. (After Weston HC. Sight, light and work, 2nd ed., Lewis London, 1962, by J. W. Grundy, 1987.)

that task. They seek to separate out misfits. The psychologist and the statistician separate out those who are successful. They are interested in finding those who have the physical skills to fit the requirements of a given task. They are interested in those who do qualify, while we are interested in discovering those who do not qualify. It is important to keep this distinction in mind. If thoroughly understood, it forms the basis for a much clearer understanding between the groups who have long needed to work more closely together, namely, statisticians and doctors (Grundy, 1981; Sheedy, 1991).

To be given sound reasons helps. One commonly stated prerequisite for a job is that vision be "adequate." The contrast in job types must be continuously kept in mind — it forms the backdrop to all our thinking.

We are now raising the question of "good vision." We are discussing a function which, in the majority of the cases, can improve via professional attention. Snell (1942) stated: "Good vision is that degree of visual function ability which is adequate to perform the visual task presented." Evidence is available to show that visual functions are important factors in safety. Thus, by bringing employees up to satisfactory visual standards, reduction of accidents will result. Kuhn (1944, 1950), Tiffin and Wirt (1945), Stump (1946), and others have studied visual skills in relation to job performance in many types of work, the results have indicated that visual skills of one sort or another are probably one of the most universal and frequent factors affecting job performance, and job performance can often be predicted, to some extent, on the basis of visual skills.

Purdue Visual Standards

The Purdue group has found that among the vision tests whose relationship with job efficiency has been extensively investigated, 12 (as previously described) have proved to be most useful.

Not only are the relationships between *individual* tests and job performance important, but the pattern of visual skills revealed by a *combination* of these twelve tests is also important. This pattern, or profile as it is called, reveals an additional relationship to job performance.

In determining the pattern of visual skills required by a job, the relationship between each of the twelve tests and performance on the job is investigated by methods Kephart (1948) discusses at length. When comparisons have been made on the basis of the individual tests, the results of all comparisons are pooled and the resulting pattern of visual skills is expressed as a battery of tests with varying cut-off scores. Not all jobs require the same pattern of visual skills.

In the 1940s the Occupational Research Center at Purdue collected data on several thousand jobs in industry, involving more than 300,000 industrial workers. Research work in many studies showed a relationship between vision and job success, revealing that there are visual skill patterns that are common to entire groups of industrial jobs.

The job profiles published in countless reports over the last five years are the result of careful and long-continued research involving large numbers of workers in a great variety of jobs. Such patterns were arrived at (statistically) by a careful observation of large numbers of statistically demonstrated relationships between test scores and job success.

Visual Job Families

Tiffin (1943) has shown that jobs differ both in the types of visual skills they demand and in the quantity of these visual skills required of the worker. Tiffin has seen further that an observation of the visual activities associated with various jobs leads us logically to suspect that such differences do exist. Controlled studies have borne out this observation.

Just as there are differences between types of jobs, however, there are also similarities between jobs. Just as we can observe differences in visual activities between such job as crane operator and radio assembler, we can observe similarities in visual activities between such jobs as lathe operator and milling machine operator. It is just as important to be aware of similarities between jobs, as it is to be aware of differences between jobs in terms of their visual requirements.

Over a number of years, the Purdue University Occupational Research Center (Tiffin and Wirt, 1945) collected data involving visual test scores and measures of job success for several thousand different industrial jobs. A careful analysis of the relationships between vision test scores and job success revealed many different job situations — groups of jobs that are similar to each other in terms of visual requirements. Within each group the visual requirements of the jobs are similar, but the requirements of each group vary from those of the next group. Thus we have a series of job groupings where the jobs within each group are essentially similar in visual requirements. This has led to the concept of *visual job families*. A visual job family is composed of a group of jobs whose visual requirements are similar.

In the 1940s, six such visual job families were identified. It is thought that the vast majority of industrial jobs will fall into one or another of these six groups in terms of the visual demands the job makes upon the worker. The visual requirements in terms of Bausch & Lomb Ortho-Rater test scores of each of the six job families, as well as further descriptions, are shown by Blais in McCunney (Blais, 2003) and in Duane (Blais, 2002) for the job families.

Kuhn (1950), on the basis of her own experience, over the period approximately from 1935 to 1950, working with industries of every description in all parts of the country and, of course, consciously and unconsciously having absorbed the philosophy developed at Purdue, has worked out minimum vision standards for use by medical directors and consultants. They are the same main profile (family) groups, but expressed in clinical terms and differing occasionally. (It is important always to remember that these are minimum.)

Eye Injuries

In 1999, Pizzarello stated that the past 50 years have seen a dramatic change in the type of eye injuries (Pizzarello, 1999). As the manufacturing sector had eroded and the workplace has changed, the nature of eye injury has also shifted. Liggett et al. (1990) found that in inner-city Los Angeles, only 8% of eye injuries occurred at work. The most common locations were in the home or on the street. Schein et al. (1988) found that 48% of injuries seen at an urban emergency room occurred at the workplace. This represents a wide discrepancy, and there is much discussion about the true extent of work-related eye injury. It is clear that many of the work-related injuries take place in auto repair and construction, as opposed to the heavy industrial setting seen in previous years. Statistics from Prevent Blindness America estimate that there are approximately 2.4 million eye injuries each year, of which approximately 250,000 or about 10% occur at the workplace. Increasingly, children are injured while at play or participating in sports. It is estimated that such injuries are in excess of 150,000 per year (Prevent Blindness America, 1996). The emphasis has therefore shifted to a more broad-based approach to eye safety. In addition, more private groups have become involved in injury prevention.

Recent developments in technology have given rise to several new areas of potential concern for eye safety. The association between video display terminals (VDT) and various forms of visual difficulty led to passage of at least one local ordinance requiring ocular evaluation of all VDT workers (Coe et al., 1980; Cole et al., 1986; Collins et al., 1998) As more data was accumulated, however, there was found to be no additional risk for such workers (Suffolk County, New York). The development of lasers led to the potential for significant ocular damage and many laser safety programs were introduced as a result. Thus, each change in technology provided new challenges to which the field of eye safety has responded effectively.

Initializing an Eye and Face Safety Program

Why Should There Be a Personal Safety Program?

Ninety-five percent of all eye injuries are preventable. Eyes, as well as other parts of the body, may be exposed to a variety of hazards in the home, in hobbies, on the farm, and in school, as well as at the worksite.

The goal of the Occupational Safety and Health Act of 1970 (OSHA, 1970), to ensure safe and healthy working conditions for working men and women in the nation, applies equally to other areas outside the workplace where the hazards may be exactly the same. The Occupational Safety and Health Act of 1970 General Duty Clause (OSHA, 1970) requires that the "employer furnish to each of his employee's employment in the place of employment which are free from recognized hazards that are causing or are likely to cause death or serious harm to his employees."

Protection of the eye from injury by physical, chemical, and radiological agents is mandatory in any occupational and safety program. To prevent an eye injury, the selection of the correct eye protective equipment, after the hazard(s) have been engineered out to the maximum extent possible, is essential.

The Cost of Blindness

There is a growing trend worldwide to evaluate disease and disability prevention on the basis of costs incurred and benefits accrued. Public health interventions to prevent blindness are particularly revealing in this respect, as cost savings and return on investment accrue, because of the avoided rehabilitative costs on the one hand, and the gains in productivity on the other.*

In 1990, the aggregated cost of blindness to the federal budget in the United States was estimated to be approximately $4.1 billion. A minimal federal budgetary cost of a person-year of blindness (vision less than 6/60 in the better eye) for a working-age adult was estimated to be $11,896.

It has been estimated that, in the U.S., if all the avoidable blindness in persons under 20 and working-age adults were prevented, a potential saving of $1 billion per year would accrue to the federal budget (Bureau of Labor Statistics, 1993).

The Cost of Eye Injuries

Anshel (1998) discussed the significant costs involved with occupational illness and injury. What most employers don't realize, however, is that there are two distinct categories of cost: The hidden costs are the costs associated with training replacement workers, property and equipment damage, missed deadlines, production delays, investigation time, overtime and downtime costs, and reduced employee attendance and morale. Research

---

* Source: World Health Organization Website 2003, Fact Sheets, February 1997, *Blindness and Visual Disability* Fact Sheet No. N145, Part IV of VII. "Socioeconomic Aspects," reproduced with the permission of the World Health Organization, © WHO/OMS, 1998, www.who.int.

TABLE 8.2

BLS Eye Injury Statistics

Benchmarks on Eye Injuries, Non-fatal Occupational Eye
Injuries, and Illnesses Involving Days Away From Work, 2000

	% Incidence of Injuries	Rate*
All private industry	3.2	5.9
Agriculture, forestry, fishing	4.0	9.8
Mining	1.9	4.6
Construction	4.2	13.4
Manufacturing	4.8	9.8
Transportation, public utilities	2.2	6.8
Wholesale trade	3.0	5.6
Retail trade	2.5	4.1
Finance, insurance, real estate	2.3	1.4
Services	2.5	3.5

* Rate of nonfatal eye injuries and illnesses per 10,000 full-time workers.

has shown that for every dollar spent on workers' compensation costs, at least four dollars are lost on hidden, often unrecorded costs.

A total of 6.8 million injuries and illnesses were reported in private industry workplaces during 1994 resulting in a rate of 8.4 cases for every 100 full time workers. Of this total of 6.8 million, nearly 6.3 million were injuries that resulted in either lost work time, medical treatment other than first aid, loss of consciousness, restriction of work or motion, or transfer to another job. The remainder of these private industry cases (about 515,000) were work-related illnesses. Employers and employees in private industry and state and local governments spent $258.5 billion for health care plans during 1992. Employer expenditures for workplace-based health care plans ($221.4 billion) were nearly six times those of employees ($37.2 billion). These numbers are expected to rise with every reporting year starting with 1992 (Bureau of Labor Statistics, 1992) (Thackery, 1982). It is easy to forget about the safety needs of workers who produce the goods and services we use everyday. Workers in industries such as construction, farming, mining and transportation still have significant injury rates.

Table 8.2 demonstrates the incidence of non-fatal occupational eye injuries and illness involving days away from work in 2000. It illustrates how eye injuries affect a variety of U.S. industries and their impact on the domestic accident burden.

An average of 2,000 eye injuries occur each day in the workplace. Ten to 20 percent of all eye injuries involve temporary or permanently disabling vision loss. Table 8.3 demonstrates the percentage distribution of numbered days away from work. This translates into disruptions in business processes and a loss of financial revenue, caused by an injury that is preventable in most cases.

TABLE 8.3

Percentage Distribution of Number of Days
Away from Work

1 day	45.2%
2 days	22.9%
3 to 5 days	20.5%
6 to 10 days	4.8%
11 to 20 days	3.1%
21 to 30 days	8.0%
31 days or more	2.6%

The costs associated with some eye and vision injuries can be estimated because of the need for treatment and workers' compensation costs, both of which are obvious costs. Within a specific workplace, the amount paid for eye injuries can be significant, especially if an eye is lost. The direct costs of a single employee losing one eye range from about $40,000 to $115,000 (Thackery, 1982). Workers' compensation laws have the loss of one eye as a scheduled benefit ranging from $5,699 to $157,685, depending on the state (U.S. Chamber of Commerce, 1989).

The MetLife demographic distribution of ear, eye, and skin ltd claims (Table 8.4) synopsizes MetLife data for the years 2001–2003.

Prevent Blindness America estimates that 3000,000 disabling eye injuries as far back as 1982 cost business and industry $330 million in lost production time, medical bills, and compensation. However, they also suggest that 90% of eye injuries are preventable.

In a study in California in 1989, the major causes of eye claims for workers' compensation were scratches and abrasions (66.8%), diseases of the eye (13.6%), burns and scalds (7.0%), cuts, lacerations, and punctures (5.1%), radiation effects (5%), infective or parasitic diseases (1.6%), and other (0.9%).

Unlike the widespread awareness of medical costs in industry, the high costs associated with untreated vision disorders are unrecognized and not easily quantifiable. These costs are found in reduced worker productivity and unnecessarily high rates of spoiled or second-class products. These costs also include the costs of accidents and co-worker injuries that could have been prevented if vision disorders had been treated. No business or industry accounts for the costs of untreated vision disorders, and therefore they are not recognized as a significant problem.

Developing an Eye Safety Program

Management dedicated to the safety and health of employees should use the program evaluation to set a standard operating procedure for personnel,

TABLE 8.4

Demographic Distribution: Eye, Ear, and Skin Ltd Claims

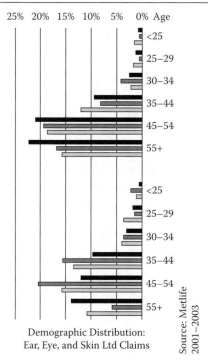

Demographic Distribution:
Ear, Eye, and Skin Ltd Claims

Source: Metlife
2001–2003

Source: Leopold, R.S., Other Diagnostic Categories — understanding otic, ophthalmic, and demographic disabilities in LTD incidence and prevalence of ear, eye and skin conditions in a year in the life of a million American workers, published by MetLife Group Disability 2003, Metropolitan Life Insurance Co., New York, New York.

and then train those employees to use, maintain, and clean the equipment to protect themselves against those hazards (OSHA, 1994).

A written personal protective equipment (PPE) program should be established for the workplace. The two basic objectives of any PPE program should be to protect the wearer from safety and health hazards, and to prevent injury to the wearer from incorrect use or malfunction of the PPE.

Steps in Developing an Eye and Safety Program

The following steps must be completed as part of and elements for developing an eye and safety program:

1. Identify hazards
2. Identify personal eye and face protection equipment (required)
3. Identify individuals exposed to the identified hazards

4. Assess hazard guidelines

5. Assign personal protective equipment to individuals for protection from hazards involved in performing their essential functions of the position

6. Provide general training prior to initiating work

7. Retrain

8. Review and evaluate the program

Identification of Hazards

Survey

Conduct a walk-through survey of the area in question. The purpose of the survey is to identify sources of all hazards, especially in this case, to the eyes and faces of workers and co-workers. The employer must certify that the hazard assessment has been completed, and a record of this certification must be retained. Consideration should be given to six basic eye and face hazard categories:

- Impact
- Heat
- Chemical
- Dust
- Optical radiation
- Contusion

Analyze Data

Having gathered and organized data on a workplace, make an estimate of the potential for eye and face injury. Each of the basic hazards should be reviewed and a determination made as to the type and level of each of the hazards found in the area. The possibility of exposure to several hazards simultaneously should be considered.

Removal of Hazardous Condition

Engineering Out Hazards

An attempt to engineer out all actual or potential hazards is the most appropriate approach to determine the hazard.

- Impose workplaces and administration controls.
- Use static shielding of equipment — barrier or deflector screens of transparent plastics can provide a clear view of a work process while protecting workers from grinding fragments, accidental sprays, or

specific optical irradiations. Cutters, grinders, and fixed-location tools have long been safeguarded by properly designed static shielding. Similarly, cathode-ray or television tubes have a radiation barrier glass over the surface exposed for viewing.

- Static shielding of personnel — physicians are familiar with the principle of static shielding in radiology offices, in which technicians or radiologists step into separate cubicles or behind leaded glass while x-ray films are exposed. Similarly, in large molten steel pours, workers now control the operation from shielded booths that protect against heat and accidental splashes. Static shielding may be suspended from the ceiling, mounted on the floor, or constructed as a separate control area.
- Utilization of PPE in conjunction with controls to limit the severity of the hazard(s) and therefore decrease the type and/or amount of PPE.

Identification of Personal Eye and Face Protection Equipment

Exactly what is PPE? Personal protective equipment includes all clothing and accessories designed to create a barrier against workplace hazards. The basic element of any PPE management program should be an in-depth evaluation of the equipment needed to protect against workplace hazards.

Appropriate PPE eye and face protective equipment is required by OSHA. OSHA mandates and their code of Federal Regulation 29 CFR 1910.133 states that eye and face protective equipment is required where there is reasonable probability of preventing injury when such equipment is used. The American National Standards Institute (ANSI) standard Z136.1-2000 is to be implemented in the prevention of laser burns, using similar engineering controls or personal protective goggles.

New ANSI Z87.1-2003

The revised ANSI Standard Z87.1-2003 American National Standard for Occupational and Educational Personal Eye and Face Protection Devices provides performance and labeling requirements for equipment designed to protect the eyes and face from physical hazards. New 2003 eye and face standards recently approved have two levels of prescription and performance:

- Basic impact
- High impact

In addition to providing testing criteria for impacts and penetration resistance, products that meet the most severe impact challenge will be marked "Z87+" on the lenses, indicating the highest level of protection.

The International Safety Equipment Association (ISEA) has published the "Use and Selection Guide for Eye and Face Protection," which is designed to assist users with the proper selection, care and maintenance of products, as well as provide information on regulations relating to eye and face protection and compliance requirements.

All frames must be tested to ensure their ability to retain a 2 mm high impact lens. New testing with high mass high velocity and penetration tends for the high impact lens. New systems of marking the lenses and frames, sideshields, have been developed.

Types of Hazards vs. PPE

Although PPE is part of the job in some industries — such as face shields for welding — as a rule, it is considered a last-resort, temporary type of protection. For normal operations, first choice will always be given to eliminating the hazard in the environment rather than using PPE (OSHA, 1994).

Assignment of PPE to Potentially Exposed

Assignment of Personal Protective Equipment to individuals for protection from hazards involved in performing their essential functions of the position. Wearing the appropriate safety eyewear is the key. Wearing safety spectacles, goggles and face shields can prevent 9 out of 10 eye injuries. Unfortunately, OSHA reports in its "Eye Protection in the Workplace Fact Sheet" that the majority of workers who sustain eye injuries in the workplace were not wearing any safety eyewear.

From material gained at the time of the visual analysis the eye protection required by the job is provided the worker. This is in the form of safety glasses that carry correcting lenses if needed and offer protection against impact through use of devices. Generally speaking, polycarbonate is the material utilized in the PPE, but case-hardened glass can be utilized if it fulfills the specific requirements. Through a single implementing device to his occupation, a twofold result is obtained, specifically, good working vision and eye protection. To prescribe the proper lenses, knowledge of the job is demanded, for occupational glasses carry with them a visual potential based on the *working distance* and a safety defense determined by the hazards characteristic of the job.

Identifying Individuals Exposed or Potentially Exposed to Identified Hazards

The area walk-through will identify the hazardous areas (OSHA, 1994). The individuals based on their job description as being actually or potentially exposed to identified hazards which cannot be engineered out or nullified by administrative controls must be identified for use of PPE.

All employees should acquire PPE appropriate for their activities/processes. Employees shall have conveniently available a type of protector suitable for the work to be performed, and they should be made to use it. No unprotected personnel are to be subjected to hazardous environment conditions. These stipulations apply also to supervisors, management personnel, and visitors while they are in hazardous areas.

Basic position(s) (e.g., electrician) duties may be changed from disassembling a motor in an atmosphere to one where the process is completed in a chemical bath. Even though the worker is still performing the electrician duties, the PPE must be changed from an impact lens to chemical goggles with or without face shield.

Personal protective equipment should be assigned to individuals for protection from hazards that result from performance of the essential functions of the position.

A summary of a questionnaire administered to patients presenting to the Massachusetts Eye and Ear Infirmary emergency services with ocular injuries in 1985 was reported by Schein (1988). All injuries were included except those due to contact lens use per se. Only 66% of all persons injured at work reported that protective eyewear was provided at the worksite. Of those suffering severe injury, only one third claimed that protective eyewear was available.

Among those injured at work, 10% stated they were wearing protective eyewear at the time of injury, and not one of these injuries was severe. Ruptured globe was the most common severe injury occurring at work. In approximately one third of the cases, a history of previous eye injury was obtained. Schein illustrated the type of eyewear worn at the time of injury for the entire study population: 70% were wearing no glasses, 10% wore safety glasses (of which 2% had side shields), 6 percent wore regular glasses, and 3% wore contact lenses. One third of the subjects whose regular glasses were broken at the time of injury suffered a severe injury.

A 1980 Bureau of Labor Statistics Study found that about 60% of workers who suffered eye injuries were not wearing eye protective equipment (Bureau of Labor Statistics, 1980). When asked why they were not wearing face protection at the time of the accident, workers indicated that face protection was not normally used in their type of work, or it was not required for the type of work performed at the time of the accident.

In a 1996 report on 8,474 cases, the United States Eye Injury Registry revealed that 78.3% of injured patients wore no protection; 3.3% wore regular spectacles. The U.S. Food and Drug Administration regulation requires that all eyeglasses and sunglasses sold to the general public be shatterproof and where the American National Standards Institute (ANSI) Z80 series standards apply; 1.8% safety glasses (ANSI Z87.1a-1991 Practice for Occupational and Educational Eye and Face Protection requirements apply).

The author was currently involved as expert witness in three lawsuits where the individual did not wear eye and face PPE or wore the wrong equipment for the hazard.

Use of Contact Lens in an Industrial Environment

The use of contact lenses at the industrial worksite has always been controversial. The question is: Are contacts dangerous? Do they worsen or lessen accidental insult from chemicals or solid foreign bodies? The dilemma is this: Should workers be permitted to wear contact lenses on the job? Should contacts be prohibited in any industrial areas and, if so, which ones? The controversy smolders because, after 25 years of rumors and misinformation, there is still a lack of hard data for employers. Much of the controversy stems from reports of serious eye injuries to workers wearing contact lenses that were incorrectly reported, never took place, or were misinterpreted. Further contributing to the controversy is the fact that during the more than 45 years since the development of the first contact lens, the type of lenses, the lens materials, and the fitting and wearing techniques have changed significantly, making it difficult to extrapolate the problems reported over the years to potential problems today.

More than 34 million Americans wear some type of contact lens. Of this number, many are employees in part of the industrial workplace. Individuals wear contact lenses for cosmetic or medical reasons; some simply prefer to wear contact lenses instead of glasses for correcting refractive errors or for visual ergonomic reasons. Contact lens wearers have sometimes been disqualified from industrial employment. Some individuals must wear contact lenses for medical reasons in order to obtain their best visual performance or efficiency and to increase their safety and proficiency in order to be able to perform the essential functions of their jobs.

Blais (1998), as Chairman of the Eye and Vision Committee of the American College of Occupational and Environmental Medicine, wrote a report regarding the status of industrial use of contact lenses. The position of national and international committees and organizations, as well as results of retrospective and prospective clinical and animal research, was summarized.

The research findings reported in this article do not reveal any direct or substantial threat associated with the use of contact lenses in hazardous ocular environments; however, in accordance with 29 CFR 1910.132, the employee must be provided and must wear the personal protective equipment required for potential hazards.

The occupational and environment medicine (OEM) physician must be able to address employee and employer concerns regarding the proper use of contact lenses in this environment. The guideline of the American College of Occupational and Environmental Medicine (ACOEM) of 2003 addresses the guidelines of the Occupational Safety and Health Administration (Blais, 2003). It is also intended to inform the occupational and environmental physician of specific standards regarding the use of contact lenses as authorized by OSHA.

OSHA Regulations

Regardless of the reason for wearing them, contact lenses do not fulfill the personal protective equipment requirements for ocular safety when worn by individuals performing eye hazardous tasks. OSHA, in the Code of Federal Regulations, requires individuals who wear contact lenses in the workplace to combine them with appropriate industrial safety eyewear.

OSHA has referenced the voluntary ANSI Z87.1 consensus standard, which makes compliance mandatory. The OSHA rule states: "The required industrial-safety eyewear for the specific hazard identified in ANSI Z87.1 must be worn over the contact lenses." Therefore, individuals who wear contact lenses are required to combine them with appropriate industrial safety eyewear (ANSI Z87.1, 2003) since contact lenses do not provide ocular protection from hazards such as particles, chemicals, and radiant energy. For example, medical personnel must wear eye and face safety devices to protect themselves from HIV or laser radiation, and cosmetologists should wear such devices to protect themselves from aerosol spray.

Zelnick et al. (1994), showed that when a respirator was worn even without spectacles, there was a loss of visual field, which varied depending on the type of full-face respirator. Since the frames of glasses have been shown to be an obstruction of the full field of vision, the combined use of a respirator plus glasses compounds the loss of visual field. "Intra mask corrections" (lenses suspended inside mask) and lenses built into a facepiece are used as a substitute for spectacles, but have poor visual ergonomics.

Individuals who wear soft contact lenses may present with symptoms of "dry eyes" due to dehydration of the contact lenses especially if there is a low blink rate. For those whose tear flow is not adequate, sometimes using artificial tears is necessary to minimize these symptoms. This may be worse in air-fed respirators but the problem is minimal in return for better visual function, work proficiency, and safety.

Challenges to federal regulations and voluntary ANSI standards which disallowed the use of contact lenses with a respirator, resulted in an OSHA-funded research project conducted by Lawrence Livermore National Laboratories (LLNL) (DaRoza, 1985). The research concluded that the "prohibition against wearing contact lenses while using a full-facepiece respirator should be revoked or withdrawn in spite of the limitations stated. Wearers of corrective lenses should have the option of wearing either contacts or eyeglasses with their full-facepiece respirators." In consideration of LLNL's research and other articles that support contact lens use, OSHA considered the prohibition unwarranted. OSHA published an enforcement procedure authorizing the use of rigid gas-permeable and soft contact lenses in all workplaces and with all types of respirators (US DOL, 1988).

Contact lenses provide the best visual ergonomics for users of full-face respirator masks. For those unable to wear contacts or those who experience problems with the contacts when using the mask (i.e., dryness), spectacles can be used. The spectacles must be of a type that will not interfere with the seal of the mask (elastic strap, intra-mask lenses).

OSHA, in paragraph (g) 1 (iii) of its preamble to Respiratory Protection rule states that "because the final standard allows contact lenses to be worn, full facepiece respirators can be worn by persons needing corrective lenses; contact lenses obviously do not interfere with facepiece seal" (CFR, 1998).

Further, the preamble of the Personal Protective Equipment (PPE) for General Industry rule states (CFR, 1994), "Based on the rule making record, OSHA believes that contact lenses do not pose additional hazards to the wearer, and has determined that additional regulation addressing the use of contact lenses is unnecessary. The Agency wants to make it clear, however, that contact lenses are not eye protective devices. If eye hazards are present, appropriate eye protection must be worn instead of, or in conjunction with, contact lenses.

Currently, OSHA statutes/rules recommend against contact lens use when working with acrylonitrile, 1,2-dibromo-3-chloropropane, ethylene oxide, methylene chloride, and 4,4-methylene dianiline chemicals. These recommendations are presumably based on best professional judgment of 1978 as no specific bases are provided in the preamble to these standards and must be adhered to until the rule is changed or a *de minimus* issued.

The 1978 National Institute for Occupational Safety and Health (NIOSH) *Pocket Guide to Chemical Hazards* recommended that workers not wear contact lenses during work with chemicals that present an eye irritation or injury hazard. This policy was recommended by the 1978 Standards Completion Program and was based on the "best professional opinion of the committee membership based on literature data" (NIOSH, 1978). The policy was also consistent at that time with general industry practice. The *NIOSH Pocket Guide 2004 Edition* contains no reference to the 1978 policy nor any discussion on contact lens in eye-hazardous environments (NIOSH, 2004).

Recommendations — ACOEM Position Statement

The following recommendations for contact lens use in an eye-hazardous environment will guide occupational safety and health professionals to safely implement the contact lens use policy.

1. *Establish a Written Policy* documenting general safety requirements for the wearing of contact lenses, including the required eye and face protection, and contact lens wear restrictions, if any, by work location or task.

2. *Conduct an Eye Hazard Evaluation* in the workplace that includes an assessment of eye-hazardous environments per OSHA Personnel Protection Standards (29 CFR 1910.132), and appropriate eye and face protection for contact lens wearers (OSHA 29 CFR 1910.133 and ANSI Z87.1-2003).

3. *Provide Training.* In addition to providing the general training required by the OSHA personal protective equipment standard (29 CFR 1910.132), provide training on employer policies on contact lens use, and first aid for contact lens wearers with a chemical exposure.

4. *Provide Personal Protective Equipment.* Comply with current OSHA regulations on contact lens wear and eye end face protection. The Code of Federal Regulations Preamble on Respiratory Protectors (29 CFR 1910.134) and Personal Protective Equipment (PPE) (CFR 1910.132) allows contact lenses to be worn under full-face respirators and other personal protective equipment for the eyes.

5. *Notify Employees and Visitors* of any denied areas where contact lenses are restricted without appropriate eye and face protection.

6. *Notify Supervisors, First Aid Responders, and EMS Responders.* Identify to supervisors and first aid responders all contact lens wearers working in eye-hazardous environments.

The Use of Multiple PPE

No single combination of protective equipment and clothing is capable of protecting against all hazards (OSHA, 1994). Thus, PPE should be used in conjunction with other protective methods. The use of PPE can itself create significant worker hazards, such as heat stress, physical and psychological stress, and impaired vision, mobility, and communication.

In general, the greater the level of PPE protection, the greater are the associated risks. For any given situation, equipment and clothing should be selected that provide an adequate level of protection. Over-protection as well as under-protection can be hazardous and should be avoided. All PPE shall be of safe design and construction for the work to be performed.

Using PPE improperly or in a manner unsuited to its design and purpose is worse than using no protection at all. Without any protection, the worker knows the worker is vulnerable and, perhaps, takes precautions. With some protection, the worker may rashly blunder into severe difficulty, thinking he or she is safe.

In ANSI Z87.1-2003 a table is published which correlates the basic types of eye hazards with the specific type of spectacle and/or face shield required for the hazard. This table will provide excellent guidance on the selection of types of eye/face safety equipment required. Although not mandated by OSHA, these requirements should be implemented when eye hazards exist in hobbies, at home, in school, in sports, or workplace where there is a reasonable probability of preventing injury when such equipment is used.

The ANSI Z87.1-2003 tables on protective devices are only representative of eye and face protective devices commonly found at the time of the writing of the standard.

General Training of Person Prior to Initiating Work

The individual must be instructed on the standard operating procedures, the limitations and benefits of each PPE, the type of potential or actual exposures, and the maintenance of the PPE. Emphasis must be made to coordinate this actual PPE with the actual hazard. If there are any deviations from the designated essential function, such that new potential hazards are incurred, the steps in the process noted heretofore must be separated (OSHA, 1994).

Where employees provide their own protective equipment, the employer shall be responsible to ensure its adequacy, including proper maintenance and sanitation of such equipment (OSHA, 1994).

Retraining

Retraining must be completed when standard operating procedures have changed, as well as the conduct of refamiliarity sessions (OSHA, 1994).

Program Review and Evaluations

How effective is the program? Is it being fully implemented? One method of measuring effectiveness is to document the injuries incurred and to review the causes and effects of deviating from the basic operating procedures.

Reassess the workplace hazard situation by identifying and evaluating new equipment and processes, reviewing accident records, and reassessing the suitability of previously selected eye and face protection (OSHA, 1994). If new hazards are present or likely to be present, the employer shall:

1. Select, and have each affected employee use, the types of PPE that will protect the affected employee from the new hazards identified in the hazard assessment.
2. Communicate selection decisions to each affected employee.
3. Select PPE that properly fits each affected employee.

Summary

The Americans with Disabilities Act (ADA) of 1990, as implemented in most facilities in July 1992 under Title 1 on employability, requires that the individual must be able to perform essential functions of the position with or without accommodation without significant risk or direct threat to themselves or to others.

OSHA mandates in the code of Federal Regulation 29 CFR 1910.133 and 1910.132 that eye and face PPE is required where there is reasonable probability of preventing injury when such equipment is used. Although not mandated by OSHA, these requirements should apply to those cases in which similar hazard exists in hobbies, at home, in school, in sports, where there is a reasonable probability of preventing injury when such equipment is used. The American National Standards Institute Z87.1-2003, on Eye and Face Protective Devices and ANSI Z136.1-2000 on Lasers sets forth the requirements on the design, construction, testing and use of the PPE devices.

In 1924, Resnick stated the following:

> The science of human rehabilitation has developed artificial hands, arms, and legs that can do almost anything the human member can do, but no one has yet produced an artificial eye that can see.... This fact alone makes the eye hazards the most serious of all non-fatal industrial accident hazards. The eye hazards...in industrial occupations still ranks second only to death in seriousness. It is true that much has been accomplished toward the alleviation of these conditions by the development of safety equipment during the last decade, particularly through the work of such organizations as the National Safety Council, the Safety Institute of America, the American Society of Safety Engineers, and the various state industrial commissions, trade associations and technical societies which have interested themselves in accident prevention and, in general, improvement of work conditions. All that has been accomplished thus far is only the beginning. (Resnick and Carris, 1924)

There is much work that needs to be completed to generate the visual standards required to perform all the eye/vision essential functions of the multiple positions and occupations available in the country.

References

American College of Occupational and Environmental Medicine (ACOEM), www.acoem.org.
Americans With Disabilities Act (ADA), 1990, Public Law, 101–336.

Birmingham Eye Trauma Terminology (BETT), Personal Communication from USEIR, Birmingham, AL, November 2001.

Blackwell, O.M. and Blackwell, H.R., Visual performance data for 156 normal observers of various ages. *J. Illum. Eng. Soc.*, 1, 3–13, 1971.

Blackwell, H.R., and Blackwell, O.M., Population data for 140 normal 20–30 year olds for use in assessing some effects of lighting upon visual performance. *J. Illum. Eng. Soc.*, 9, 158–174, 1980.

Blais, B.R., Visual Ergonomics of the Workplace, Presented at the American Occupational Health Conference, May 23, 1994.

Blais, B.R., Basics of Occupational Ophthalmology, Volume 5, Chapter 37. In: Tasman, W., Jaeger, EA (eds), *Duane's Clinical Ophthalmology.* Philadelphia: Lippincott Williams Wilkins, 2002.

Blais, B.R., Tredici, T.J., and Williams, J., Occupational Ophthalmology, Chapter 34. In: McCunney R (ed), *A Practical Approach to Occupational and Environmental Medicine. 3rd Edition.* Philadelphia: Lippincott Williams Wilkins, April 2003.

Blais, B.R., Eye Chapter 16 ACOEM Occupational Medicine Practice Guidelines, Beverly Hills, Mass, OEM Press. 2003, December 2nd Edition.

Boyce, P.R., and Simons, R.H., Hue discrimination and light sources, *Ltg. Res. Technol.* 9, 125–140, 1977.

Brownell, C.P., Visual fact-finding discloses relationship of visual capacity and job performances, *Safety Engineering* 93: 24–26, 48–49, April 1947.1

Bureau of Labor Statistics: Report #597, Washington, DC, Bureau of Labor Statistics, 1980.

Bureau of Labor Statistics, Expenditures for health care plans by employers and employees, 1992. Press Release.

Code of Federal Regulations — Parts 1900 to 1910 Respiratory Protection, 29 CFR 1910.134 (e) (5) (ii), Revised July 1990.

Code of Federal Regulations — Parts 1910 Personal Protection Equipment for General Industry. Final Rule, CFR 29.1910.132 effective July 5, 1994, Fed Reg. Vol. 59, no. 66. Wednesday. April 6, 1994 Rules and Regulations pp 16343. www.osha.gov/pls/oshaweb/owadisp.show_document? p_table=PREAMBLES &p id=1022&p text version=FALSE

Code of Federal Regulations — Parts 1910 and 1926 Respiratory protection final rule. Fed Reg. Vol. 63. no. 5. Thursday, January 5, 1998 Rules and Regulations p. 1162. www.osha.gov/pls/ oshaweb/owadisp.show_document?p_table = PREAMBLES & p id=1022&p text version=FALSE.

Coe, J.V., Cuttle, K., McClellan, W.C., et al., Visual Display Units: A Review of Potential Health Problems Associated with Their Use, Wellington, New Zealand Department of Health Regional Unit, 1980.

Cole, B.L., Breadon, I.D., Sharp, K., et al., Comparison of the Symptoms Reported by VDT Users and Non-VDT Users, Bulletin No. 2, Melbourne, University of Melbourne, 1986.

Collins, M.I., Brown, B., and Bowman, K.J., Visual Discomfort and VDTs, Queensland, Centre for Eye Research, Department of Optometry, Queensland Institute of Technology, 1998.

DaRoza, R.A., Weaver C: Is it safe to wear contact lenses with a full facepiece respirator? Berkeley, CA: Lawrence Livermore National Laboratory (UCRL - 53653). August 16, 1985.

EEOC, Equal Employment Opportunity Commission, *Americans with Disabilities Handbook*, Section 1630.2(m), 1992.

EEOC, Equal Employment Opportunity Commission, Technical Manual, Title 1, ADA, January 1992 Rehabilitation Act.

Grundy, J.W., Visual efficiency in industry. *Ophthal. Optician*, 21, 548–552, 1981.

Grundy, J.W., When your car could break down through a visual defect. *Ophthal. Opt.*, Feb 4, 77–80, 1984.

Grundy, J.W., A simple method of occupational vision requirements. *Optom. Today*, Oct 11, 684–688, 1986.

Grundy, J.W., A diagrammatic approach to occupational optometry and illumination. *Optom. Today*, Aug 1, 503–508, 1987.

Grundy, J.W., Prescribing and patient management: occupational and recreational considerations. *Optometry*, K. Edwards and R. Llewellyn (eds), Butterworths, London, 1988.

Harris, J., Foundations of Occupational Medicine Practices Prevention, Chapter 1, *Occupational Medicine Guidelines*. Glass, L. (ed), OEM Press. Edition 2, 2003.

Julian, W.G., Variation in near visual acuity with illuminance for a group of 27 partially sighted people. *Ltg. Res. Technol.*, 16, 34–41, 1984.

Keeney, A., The Eye and the Workplace: Special Considerations, *Duane's Clinical Ophthalmology*, W. Tassman, M.D., E. Jaeger, M.D. (eds), Lippincott, Philadelphia, PA, p. 199.

Kephart, N.C., An example of increased production through an industrial vision program, *Opt. J. & Rev.* September 15, 1948.

Koven, A.L., The right eyes for the right job. *TAAOO*, Sept/Oct 1947, 46–52.

Kuhn, H., Transactions of the American Academy of Ophthalmology and Otolaryngology, December 1946.

Kuhn, H., Transactions of the American Academy of Ophthalmology and Otolaryngology, July/August 1941.

Kuhn, H.S., *Industrial Ophthalmology*, St. Louis: Mosby, 1944.

Kuhn, H.A., *Eyes and Industry*, St. Louis: CV Mosby, 1950.

Liggett, P.E., Pince K.I., Barlow, W., Ocular trauma in an urban population, *Ophthalmology*, 97:581, 1990.

North, R.V., *Work and the Eye*, Oxford University Press, Oxford, 1993.

OSHA, Williams-Steiger Occupational Safety and Health Act of 1970 (OSHA). 84 Stat 1593.

OSHA 29CFR 1910.132. Personal Protective Equipment. OSHA 3077.1994, rev. Washington, DC, Occupational Safety and Health Administration, 1994.

OSHA 29CFR 1910.133. Occupational and Educational Rehabilitation Act of 1973, Section 50429 USG para. 794.

Pizzarello, L., Eye safety and the economic impact of eye injuries, during the last century in the United States, *Sports and Industrial Ophthalmology*, 12(3), September 1999.

Pocket Guide to Chemical Hazards. National Institute for Occupational Safety and Health. 1978 edition.

Pocket Guide to Chemical Hazards. National Institute for Occupational Safety and Health. 2004 edition.

Prevent Blindness America: Summary materials, Schaumburg, IL: Prevent Blindness America, 1996.

Resnick, L., Carris, L.H., Eye Hazards in Industrial Occupations. National Committee for the Prevention of Blindness, NY, 1924.

Riggs, L.A., Visual acuity. In *Vision and Visual Perception*. Graham, C.H. (ed), Wiley, New York, 1965, pp. 321–349.

Schein, O.D., Hibbard, P.L., Shingleton, B.J., The spectrum and burden of ocular injury. *Ophthalmology*, 95:300–305, 1988.

Sheedy, J.E., *Vision and Computer Displays, 2nd ed.*; Vision Analysis: Walnut Creek, CA, 1991.

Silver, J.H., Gould, E.S., Irvine, D., and Cullinan, T.R., Visual acuity at home and in eye clinics. *Ophthal. Optician*, 20, p. 4, 1980.

Snell, A.C., The need for more realistic ophthalmic service in industry. *NYS Journal of Medicine* 42:1435, 1942.

Stump, N.F., How inefficient vision causes industrial accidents. *The Optometric Weekly*, July 4, 1946.

TAAOO, Transactions of the American Academy of Ophthalmology and Otolaryng-ology, July/August 1941, National Society for the Prevention of Blindness, p. 30.

TAAOO, Transactions of the American Academy of Ophthalmology and Otolaryng-ology, November/December 1942, p. 131, AAOO Council Minutes.

TAAOO, Transactions of the American Academy of Ophthalmology and Otolaryng-ology, Business Meeting Committee of Industrial Ophthalmology, 10 Oct. 1942, p. 143.

TAAOO, Transactions of the American Academy of Ophthalmology and Otolaryng-ology, Announcements, Industrial Ophthalmology, March/April 1943, p. 315.

TAAOO, Transactions of the American Academy of Ophthalmology and Otolaryng-ology, January/February 1944, Business Meeting of the Joint Industrial Oph-thalmology Committee, p. 105.

TAAOO, Transactions of the American Academy of Ophthalmology and Otolaryng-ology, Supplement, June 1944, pp. 1–8.

Thackery, J. The high cost of workplace eye trauma: The 90% avoidable injury. *Sightsaving Magazine*, 51(1), 19–22, 1982.

Tiffin, J., Wirt, E.D., Determining visual standards for industrial jobs by statistical method. *Am Acad Ophthalmol Otolaryngol* 58:4, 1945.

Tiffin, J., *Visual Skills and Vision Tests, Industrial Psychology*, New York: Prentice Hall, 1943.

US Chamber of Commerce (1989) Analysis of Workers' Compensation Laws. Wash-ington, DC: US Chamber of Commerce.

US District Court Stipulation of Settlement, RE Keith, *B. Kimble, et al. v. Dr. George Hayes et al.*, May 2, 1992.

US DOL Memorandum to Regional Administrators Regarding Contact Lenses Used with Respirators, 29 CFR 1910.34 (5) (ii), February 1988.

Verriest, G., Vandevyvere, R., and Vanderdonck, R. Nouvelles reserches se rapportant a líinfluence du sexe et de líage sur la discrimination chromatique ainsi quía la signification practique des resultants du test 100 hue de Farnsworth-Munsell. *Res. DíOptique*, 41, p. 499, 1962.

Westheimer, G., Visual acuity. In *Adler's Physiology of the Eye* (8th ed.), CV Mosby, St. Louis, 1987, pp. 415–428.

Zelnick, S.O., McKay, R.T., and Lockey, J.E., Visual field loss while wearing fullface respirator protection. *Am Ind Hyg Assoc J*. April 1994; 55:315–321.

9

Kids and Computers

Alan Hedge

CONTENTS

Computer Use by Children and Adolescents

In the U.S., the use of a computer has become an integral part of the daily activities of many children. In schools children use computers for educational purposes in their classrooms, laboratories, and libraries. Federal and state government have pushed for the widespread introduction of computers in schools. For example, in 2002 the state of Maine initiated a program, the Maine Learning Technology Initiative,* to equip all 7th and 8th grade public school students and teachers across the state with portable computers. A U.S. Department of Education survey, mailed to a representative sample of

---

* http://www.state.me.us/mlte/

1,209 public schools in the 50 states and the District of Columbia, reported that, in the fall of 2001, 99% of public schools in the United States had access to the Internet, and 85% of schools had a broadband connection (Kleiner and Farris, 2002). The ratio of students to instructional computers with Internet access in public schools was 5.4 to 1 in 2001, compared with a 12.1 to 1 ratio in 1998. School children were allowed Internet access outside of regular school hours in 51% of the public schools surveyed, and this was more prevalent among secondary schools (78%) than elementary schools (42%). Similarly, Internet access outside of regular school hours was more common-place in large schools with enrollments of 1000 students or more (82%) than medium-sized and small schools (47%), and of these schools, 95% made Internet access available after school, 74% before school, and 6% on week-ends.

In today's information-driven world the goal of such educational initia-tives is to make the computer a ubiquitous tool for the teacher and the learning child. A September 2001 survey gathered interview data from about 56,000 households and collected information regarding 28,002 5- to 17-year-old children, including those enrolled in school and those not enrolled in school. Results showed that computers were used by around 90% (47 million persons) and about 59% (31 million persons) used the Internet (DeBell and Chapman, 2003). This survey also found that at every age range computer use was more prevalent at school (81%) than at home (65%) (see Figure 9.1).

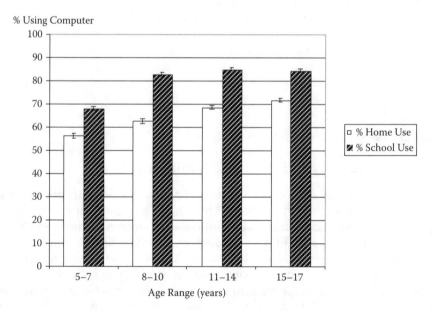

FIGURE 9.1
Computer use in school and at home by children and adolescents ages 5 to 17 years (redrawn from DeBell and Chapman, 2003).

At home, many children use a computer for entertainment, for educational purposes, and as the most common location to connect to the Internet. DeBell and Chapman (2003) also found that a home computer was used by 59% of 5- through 17-year-olds to play games, 46% use it to connect to the Internet, and 44% used a home computer to complete school assignments. Of those who used the Internet, about 72% used it to complete school assignments, 65% used it for e-mail or instant messaging, and 62% used it to play games.

Rideout et al. (2003) conducted a nationally representative random-digit-dial telephone survey of 1,065 parents of children ages six months through six years in the U.S.A. They found that 31% of 0- to 3-year-olds and 70% of 4- to 6-year-olds had used a computer. In combination, the results showed that 48% of children ages 6 years and younger had used a computer at home. When asked about the amount and proficiency of computer use by 4- to 6-year-olds, results showed that on a typical day 27% spent an average of 1 h 4 min at the keyboard, 39% used a computer several times a week or more, 37% could turn the computer on by themselves, and 40% could load a CD-ROM.

Internationally, there is some variability in the pattern of computer use in developed countries and this may reflect climate and socioeconomic factors. Vryzas, and Tsitouridou (2002) surveyed a random sample of 993 children, 305 of whom had a home computer that was primarily used for games. In contrast, a 2002 survey of 5,400 school children in Finland found that 20% of boys, aged 13 to 15 years, used a computer more than 3 h a day, and that home computer use was even greater in Denmark, Estonia, Norway, and Sweden (Currie et al., 2004).*

When this amount of computer use is combined with other manually intensive uses of the hands, such as is required when children play handheld videogames or when they send text messages on a cellular telephone, there may be a greater potential for accelerating the onset of a musculoskeletal disorder, either later in childhood or earlier in adulthood. We do not gather national statistics on the incidence and prevalence of musculoskeletal injuries among children and so we cannot assess the degree to which such injuries may be changing as a consequence of the widespread use of information technologies. However, such data have been gathered for adults and the findings from numerous research studies suggest a possible association between computer use and upper body musculoskeletal disorders (MSDs) arising from the cumulative amount of repetitive, forceful, stressful hand movements required to perform work, such as is involved in intensive use of a keyboard and mouse, and the posture of the hands (see for example, NRC-IOM, 2001). Children in modern societies are being increasingly exposed to computer use, and it is quite possible that this will increase the risks of musculoskeletal injuries unless appropriate ergonomic guidelines are followed (Straker, 2001). The lack of funding for the research necessary for developing accurate and valid ergonomic design guidelines for computer

---

* http://e.finland.fi/netcomm/news/showarticle.asp?intNWSAID=26581

use may result in the unintentional scarring of a whole generation of school children by increasing their susceptibility to developing MSDs (Straker, Harris and Zandvliet, 2000).

Computers and CVS Risks in Children and Adolescents

Computer use has been linked to computer vision syndrome (CVS), which is the complex of eye and vision-related problems, such as eyestrain, blurred vision, dry and irritated eyes, tired eyes, and headaches, that have been associated with computer use (Anshel, 1998). Studies of adult computer use have shown that CVS is significantly associated with the daily hours of computer use (Hedge, 1991). CVS has also been shown to be more prevalent in workplaces illuminated with direct, downlighting systems, such as those found in schools, compared with indirect, uplighting systems (Hedge, Sims and Becker 1995). Unfortunately, to date there has been relatively little research on these topics with children, but the few studies that have been conducted suggest that we should expect a similar association between computer use and CVS.

Marumoto et al. (1996) investigated whether sitting posture is associated with the failing eyesight of young students while studying at a computer. They found that the viewing distance of myopic children was significantly shorter than that of the normal-sighted children, and the average viewing distance of the 10 myopes studied was 15.0 cm, which is extremely short given the generally recommended viewing distance of 50 to 70 cm for computer screen operation that is derived from the resting position of the eye. They found that viewing distance was significantly correlated with the neck flexion angle, viewing angle, near-point, and accommodative power. They also showed that the shorter viewing distance while studying created postural problems, such as extreme neck flexion, which also decreased the accommodative power of the eyes and exacerbated failing eyesight of young students. In a subsequent study, Marumoto et al., (1999) conducted a more detailed investigation of how the posture of 19 13-year-old students was related to degradation of vision. When the students were studying printed materials a significant relationship between viewing distance and eye accommodation, near point (cm), viewing angle, and neck angle was demonstrated, and they concluded that poor posture, particularly decreased neck angle, is significantly related to the degradation of vision in children.

A field study of office workers investigated the preferred position of computer visual displays relative to the eyes, how this affected reports of visual strain, and whether there were any systematic individual differences in screen arrangement (Jaschinski, Heuer, and Kylian, 1998). Results showed that those working at high screens (screen center at eye level) reported greater eyestrain than those with lower screens (screen center 18 cm below eye level). When free to adjust screen distance, the most comfortable and preferred screen position was placement this at a viewing distance between 60 and 100 cm and at a 16-degree downwards vertical inclination of gaze. More visual strain was reported when forced to work at a shorter viewing distance.

Computers and MSD Risks in Children and Adolescents

Musculoskeletal disorders (MSDs) are soft-tissue injuries of connective tissues (tendon, tendon sheath, ligament, and fascia), muscles, or nerves (e.g., carpal tunnel syndrome is caused by median nerve compression). Computer use is also associated with vision problems (computer vision syndrome). Table 9.1 gives a summary of the most common types of MSDs and vision problems reported by adults that appear to be associated with prolonged work time at a computer where little attention has been paid to improving the ergonomic design of the workplace.

Numerous studies have been conducted on the etiology of musculoskeletal disorders (e.g., Armstrong et al., 1993; Buckle and Devereux, 1999; Kumar, 2001; NRC-IOM, 2001) and these have shown that injury risks are influenced by a variety of individual factors (e.g., genetics, age, gender, anthropometry); physical environment and biomechanical factors (e.g., force, strength, posture, cold, vibration); and task demands (e.g., repetitive paced tasks, stress). Although most children do not yet use computers with the sustained intensity of adults, the body of the developing child generally is smaller and weaker than that of an adult. Consequently, if children are exposed to those factors known to increase injury risks in adults, then it is possible that this exposure may accelerate the subsequent onset of an injury. Moreover, if it is found that children are being exposed to unnecessary risk factors, then we should strive to both improve the design of the environments in which they use computers and to educate them on the appropriate and safe use of computers so that they develop lifelong protective skills that will carry into adulthood and continue to protect them when in the world of work.

To date there has been only a small number of ergonomic research studies of computer use by school children, but the results obtained from this work suggest that possible adverse health effects might arise from extended computer use on inappropriately designed school furniture. Oates, Evans and Hedge (1998) investigated computer use among 95 elementary school children (46 boys, 49 girls) in 3rd, 4th and 5th grades (ages 8.5 to 11.5 years) randomly sampled from three school settings: an urban, a suburban, and a rural school. The stature of each child was measured and results showed that the selected sample was comprised of approximately equal numbers of pupils at the 5th, 50th, and 95th percentiles for stature. In each school, the researchers observed children working on a novel text-writing task using a

TABLE 9.1

Summary of the Most Common Upper Limb Musculoskeletal Disorders and Vision Problems Possibly Associated with Adult Computer Use

MSD	Affected Area	Cause	Symptoms
Tendonitis	Wrist, hand	Irritation or inflammation of the tendon caused by repeated microtrauma	Discomfort, ache, pain at the tendon that is amplified by awkward and/or forceful movements.
Tenosynovitis	Wrist, hand	Irritation or inflammation of the tendon sheath caused by repeated microtrauma	Discomfort, ache, pain at the tendon sheath that is amplified by awkward and/or forceful movements.
Epicondylitis	Elbow	Over use or strain of the muscles attached to the bone at this part of the elbow which become inflamed, swollen, painful and tender to touch	Outer part of the elbow is painful and tender (lateral epicondylitis — "Tennis elbow"). Inner part of the elbow is painful and tender to touch (medial epicondylitis — "Golfer's elbow").
Carpal tunnel syndrome	Wrist	Median nerve compression, neuropathy	Hand pain in the night. Hand numbness and or pins and needles, affecting the thumb, first, second and half of the third finger nearest to the thumb. Weakness of some thumb movements; wasting of the muscles at the base of the thumb. Pain in the lower end of forearm.
Cubital tunnel syndrome	Elbow	Ulnar nerve compression, neuropathy	Pain, swelling, weakness, or clumsiness of the hand and tingling or numbness of the third and fourth fingers. Elbow pain on the side of the arm next to the chest.
Computer Vision syndrome	Eyes	Fatigue of the extraocular and intraocular muscles; low blink rate, dryness of eyes	Sore, irritated, tired eyes, difficulties in focusing, blurry vision, headaches.

desktop computer in their typical computer work area. The dimensions and layout of the workspace and the school furniture were recorded. After 5 minutes of observation, the working posture of each child was evaluated using a validated ergonomic posture targeting method, the rapid upper limb

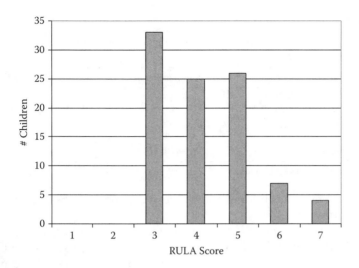

FIGURE 9.2
Postural Risk Assessments for in 3rd, 4th, and 5th grade schoolchildren using a computer for word processing (redrawn from Oates et al., 1998).

assessment (RULA) method (McAtamney and Corlett, 1993). This method estimates the risk of a musculoskeletal injury based upon the awkwardness of the working posture. A total score of 2 or less indicates an acceptable ergonomic design; a score of 3 or 4 indicates that further investigation is needed and changes in the design are required; a score of 5 or 6 indicates that further investigation and changes are required very soon; and a score of 7 indicates that further investigation and changes are required immediately. The results obtained by Oates et al. (1998) are shown in Figure 9.2 and from this it is obvious that none of the children were using a computer in an ideal arrangement and that the RULA scores for many children placed them in a very poor posture that put them into the "at risk of injury" categories. Indeed, 61% fell in the 3 to 4 range, 35% fell in the 5 to 6 range, and 4% were scored at a 7.

The poor postures that were observed resulted from several factors: the computer keyboards were used on flat surfaces that were too high for the seated dimensions of the children; the computer keyboards often were sloped upwards thereby creating deviated wrists that were bent upwards when the child typed; the computer monitors were placed much too high causing the children to bend their necks backwards; and the work surface heights and chair designs were unsuitable for the anthropometric dimensions of the children — many children worked with their legs and feet dangling (see Table 9.2).

Thankfully, in these schools the duration of computer work often was relatively short, and this helps to minimize any adverse effects of poor posture on injury risks. However, as computer use becomes more intense both at school and at home, the consequences of these mismatches between

TABLE 9.2

Comparison of Observed and Recommended Dimensions for Workstation Furniture for School Computer Use

Workstation Dimension	Recommended	Observed
Computer keyboard height	21.5–24"	25.6–39.4"
Computer monitor height	31.5–38"	37.4–51.2"
Chair backrest height	26–30"	23.6–31.5"
Chair seat pan width	13–15"	11.8–17.7"
Chair back rest angle	90°–120°	90°–108°

Source: Oates et al. (1998) *Computers in the Schools*, 14, 3/4, 55–63.

the furniture and the children and the resulting poor postures may become more serious.

Straker et al. (2000) conducted two studies on children's computers use. In their first study they investigated computer use in 24 schools in Canada and Australia. In these schools, they assessed both the physical and psychosocial environments, and 1404 students completed a survey questionnaire. They found that many children rated the physical aspects of their computer workstations as being poorly designed. Their second study investigated three Australian schools with mandatory laptop programs and they found that 60% of students reported musculoskeletal discomfort when using their laptops.

Kleiner and Farris (2002) found that in 2001, 10% of public schools lent laptop computers to students and that 53% of these schools lent laptop computers for 1 week or more. Of these schools, 22% lent laptops to children for the entire school year. In 2004, the Varina School District, outside of Richmond, VA, purchased more than 23,000 laptop computers for their entire school district. This is the first known instance where an entire school district is using computers as their sole educational instrument. However, laptops are not ergonomically designed because the screen and keyboard are attached so that when the screen is at a comfortable height and distance, the keyboard usually isn't and vice versa. Consequently, several studies have investigated the effects of laptop computer use by children.

The physical impact of computer use on upper body posture and on muscle activity has been studied in 32 school-aged children (20 boys and 17 girls aged 4 to 17 years old) while sitting on a standard school chair at a standard school desk and while reading from a book, from a laptop computer, and from a desktop computer (Straker, Briggs and Greig, 2002; Briggs, Straker and Greig, 2004). Surface electromyography (EMG) data on the activity in the left and right upper back muscles (cervical erector spinae and upper trapezius muscles) were recorded and results showed that there was greater activity with laptop use than with reading from a book or with using a desktop computer. Children were videotaped and the images were digitized to analyze a series of body angles: head tilt, neck flexion, trunk flexion, and gaze angle. They found that seated posture was significantly different for

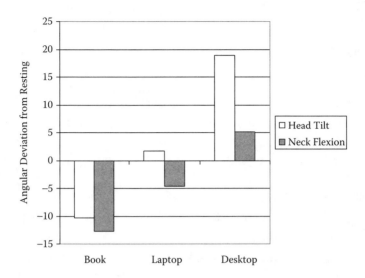

FIGURE 9.3
Postural differences in reading a book, reading from a laptop computer, and reading from a desktop computer (Briggs et al., 2004). (Note: Negative values indicate increased head tilt and neck flexion; positive values indicate decreased head tilt and neck flexion.)

reading a book and computer use, and that book use was the worst for forward tilt of the head and for neck flexion; laptop use involved less head tilt and neck flexion, and that use of a desktop computer resulted in the best reading posture with the head most vertical and the neck not flexed (see Figure 9.3). Overall, children adopted the best posture when working at a desktop computer.

The effects of using a laptop computer have been studied in a survey of 314 Australian children, aged 10 to 17 years, along with detailed interviews and observation of 20 other children who were using laptop computers. Results showed that mean daily laptop use was 3.2 h, mean weekly laptop use was 16.9 h. The postures adopted for laptop use were highly varied as a function of location of use (e.g., home, school, and boarding house), and 60% of children reported postural discomfort that was correlated with time of use per session, rather than days of use (Harris and Straker, 2000).

Guidelines for Using Computers

One way to decrease the possible risks of computer use is to educate children in appropriate computer ergonomics. Ergonomists generally agree that working in a neutral posture minimizes musculoskeletal injury risks. For computer use, achieving a neutral posture involves:

- Upper and lower back well supported by chair that allows some back recline
- Chair height adjusted so that the seat does not compress the knees or thighs
- Feet firmly planted on a surface for support (either the floor or a footrest)
- Head balanced on neck (not tilted backward or too far forward, not bent or twisted)
- Upper arms close to body and relaxed (not abducted to the side or flexed forward)
- Sitting so that the:
  - Angle formed by the shoulders, hips, and knees is >90 degrees
  - Angle formed by the shoulder, elbow, and wrist is >90 degrees
  - Angle formed by the hips, knees, and feet is >90 degrees
  - Wrists at a neutral position, level with forearm (<15 degrees deviation)

Although children have the same postural needs as adults when it comes to computer use, they also have some unique needs. Appropriate adjustability of furniture and equipment is absolutely essential when a family shares a computer workstation. A child, especially a very young one, may not be very aware of the position of his/her extremities in space and they may not attend to postural discomfort and minor aches and pains, so it is especially important for an adult to monitor their computer use and correct any posture problems that are observed. Children may respond more to images than to writing when it comes to learning about the ideal workstation posture. Adults should try showing them "before" and "after" pictures of workstations. Children, especially the younger ones, have smaller hands than adults and they have less strength. A conventional-size keyboard may be too large for comfortable use, so choosing appropriately sized equipment is important. Sometimes children like to use trackballs instead of mice because their small hands find them easier to handle. A small mouse may be just as good. Being able to adjust chairs, monitors, and desks is important, and children should be taught how to make appropriate adjustments in order to be comfortable. With younger children, these adjustments may need to be made by an adult. Be sure that children understand and are physically strong enough to make adjustments (some mechanisms are even difficult for adults). Finally, children may find it more difficult than adults to know when to take breaks from typing or surfing the Web, and thus it is helpful to monitor how long a child has been using a computer.

To encourage children to work in neutral postures, some schools are beginning to institute ergonomics programs to educate students, teachers, and parents on ways to reduce the risks of computer-related musculoskeletal injuries. Barrero and Hedge (2000) and Saito et al. (2000) have formulated comprehensive ergonomics guidelines for the parents of school children and for schools that can be incorporated as part of such an ergonomics program. All ergonomic guidelines for computer use focus on preventing musculo-skeletal injury by trying to keep the user's body posture in neutral positions while using the computer. Ergonomic guidelines have been formulated to provide guidance on appropriate configurations for computer workstation furniture. In this chapter, these two sets of guidelines have been integrated to create the following guidelines for safe computer use.

Work Environment and Workstation Layout

The goal is to "create an environment that fits the work of the child." To do this you should:

- Verify that the environment is appropriate for computer work. Appropriate environmental conditions are:
  - Illumination 300 to 500 lux (horizontal plane)
  - Temperature 24 to 27° C in summer, 20 to 23°C in winter
  - Humidity 50 to 60%
  - Noise Level 55 dB(A) or less
- There should be no glare on the computer screen. If you can see glare, then reposition the screen until it is glare-free, but check that the viewing angle is still comfortable. If repositioning alone does not work, use a good-quality, glass, anti-glare screen. If left uncorrected, glare will cause discomfort, eyestrain, and headaches. Make sure that the computer is in a location that is neither too bright nor too dark. To avoid possible problems with daylight, make sure that windows have blinds or drapes to regulate daylight levels. Avoid positioning the computer screen so that it either faces or backs to a bright window. Avoid very glossy work surfaces and furnishings, such as mirrors and shiny metal, which can contribute to glare. The noise level should be comfortable and not uncomfortably loud because this can cause stress, which in turn causes the muscles to tense which may accelerate a musculoskeletal injury. Make sure that the room is well ventilated, with adequate heating and cooling to minimize thermal discomfort.
- Make sure that there is enough space on the desk for the computer screen, keyboard, mouse, or other input device, as well as paper documents and any other components that are required.

Working Posture

The goal is to "avoid unnatural postures, and change your posture occasionally." To achieve this it is necessary to:

- Make sure that everything to be used is within the normal working area, including books, documents, tools, a telephone, etc. The normal work area corresponds to the space and objects that can be reached by a person while sitting in front of a computer, without having to twist the body or reach far.
- If the child has to type materials from a book or document, then make sure that the printed copy is placed in a document holder that is placed near the screen, in order to avoid head twisting.
- If most of the computer work being performed involves keyboard use, then make sure that the body is centered on the alphanumeric part of the keyboard (align the center of the body with the H key), because most keyboards are asymmetrical in design (the alphanumeric keyboard is to the left and a numeric keypad to the right).
- Avoid staying in postures where you are bent too far forward or backward, or twisted for an extended period of time.

The following sections provide information on the best positions for using a keyboard, mouse, or other input device and computer screen; on the features to look for in an ergonomic chair; and on appropriate patterns of working at a computer.

Work Surface

The goal is to "provide a stable work surface that comfortably fits the dimensions of the child." Be sure that the surface is large enough to support all of the needed materials, even those that are not currently being used. In particular you should:

- Make sure that the computer screen, keyboard, mouse, or other input device is on a stable work surface that doesn't shake or wobble. If children and adults will use the same work surface, then choose either a split-height adjustable work surface, where the rear surface adjusts to position the computer screen and the front surface adjusts to position the keyboard, mouse etc., or a support surface that has some overall height adjustability, or best of all a height-adjustable, negative-slope keyboard tray that can help to keep the elbows open at a >90 degrees angle and that will allow the wrists to remain in a neutral position while typing (see Figure 9.4).
- Check that there is enough space underneath the desk for free leg movement.

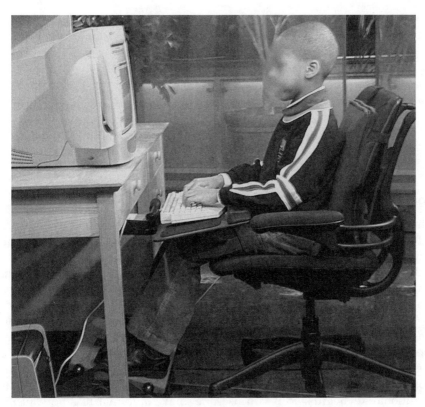

FIGURE 9.4
Neutral posture for desktop computer use by a 6-year-old boy. (Photograph from the Today Show, January 5, 2000.) http://ergo.human.cornell.edu/Todayimages/Sheldonl2.jpg

Chair

The goal is to "provide a chair that matches the size of the child for comfortable sitting." The more adjustments there are on a chair, the greater the number of people that should be able to comfortably sit on it. However, if only one person is using the chair and it feels comfortable to that person, then the degree of adjustability will be less important. To find a suitable chair you should:

- Use an ergonomic chair that positions the child so that his or her forearms are about parallel in height to the keyboard. Achieving this position may require using a chair with adjustable seat height.
- With the chair height adjusted, the child's feet should either be flat on the floor, or if not, then the child should be provided an adjustable footrest (see Figure 9.4).

- Use an ergonomic chair with back adjustment features, especially height adjustable lumbar support. If the back tension of the chair back does not adjust, then make sure that the lower back is firmly supported in some way.

- If the chair has armrests, then make sure that they are height-adjustable: The best armrests will allow you to rest the area of your forearm that lies halfway between your wrist and elbow, without compressing any part of the arm. Look for armrests that are broad, flat, and cushioned.

Keyboard

The goal is to "position the keyboard at a desirable angle to put the hands into a neutral posture, and use a palm rest if necessary." Most ergonomic keyboards on the market today are split keyboards (those where the alphanumeric keys are split at an angle). These keyboards mainly address the problem of wrist ulnar deviation (side-to-side bending of the hands). However, wrist extension and flexion (vertical movement of the hands bending up and down) are more important for musculoskeletal injury prevention. There is no consistent research that shows that ergonomic split keyboards alone will provide the optimal postural benefits, and for most people a regular keyboard design works just fine if it's placed in the proper neutral position. Some people find split keyboards to be more comfortable than traditional keyboards, so if you use one, make sure that it is not causing your shoulders to abduct away from the body or be raised higher than is comfortable. To achieve a neutral hand/wrist position when using a keyboard you should:

- Use the flattest keyboard that you can find (modern keyboards are getting flatter and flatter). If you have an upward sloping keyboard then make sure that the rear feet on the keyboard are not extended. The flatter the keyboard, the less you have to bend your wrist upwards during typing. This upward position can increase the risk of a hand/wrist injury such as carpal tunnel syndrome.

- Place the keyboard on a height-adjustable, negative-slope keyboard tray. The negative slope provides a downward tilt to the surface on which the keyboard sits, and this in turn flattens out the keyboard with respect to the hands (see Figure 9.4).

- Make sure there is space in front of the keyboard for you to comfortably rest your hands (this space can be on the desktop surface itself if the keyboard is thin). Look for a flatter, firm but not hard, wide, and deep palm support and rest the base of the palm of the hands in between bursts of typing activity to give the hands some rest time in a neutral position.

- If you are using a laptop computer and the keyboard seems difficult to use, then use an external keyboard, preferably one that is placed on a negative-slope keyboard tray.

Nonkeyboard Input Devices

The goal is to "use a pointing device that is comfortable, easy to use, and that puts your hand and forearm in a neutral position." There is no conclusive research that says that one type of pointing device (mouse, trackball, stylus, touch pad, joystick, etc.) is better for you than another. Just make sure that when you use a pointing device, whether it's a mouse, trackball, touchpad, multitouch pad, or joystick, that whatever you use feels comfortable, fits your hand, and allows you to work in a neutral hand and body posture. To achieve a neutral hand/wrist position when using a nonkeyboard input device you should:

- Choose a nonkeyboard input device, such as a mouse, trackball, or touchpad, that feels comfortable to use and that puts the hand in the most neutral position possible.
- If you use a mouse, choose an optical mouse rather than a mechanical roller-ball mouse, because this will have less resistance to movement and will not require cleaning.
- If the nonkeyboard input device has buttons, make sure that these are comfortably positioned under your fingers and thumb and that they do not require too much force to use.
- Use a height-adjustable, gliding support platform that allows the mouse to be positioned close to the side of the body, and to the side of or immediately above the keyboard tray (so that the arm does not have to reach to the side).

Display

The goal is to "provide a glare-free screen that can be comfortably seen by adjusting the display's height, tilt angle, brightness, contrast, and other settings." This goal can be achieved by ensuring that:

- The computer screen is height and angle adjustable and adjusted to the position that works best. Adjust the display angle so that light sources such as ceiling lights, task lights, and windows are not reflected on the display. Slightly tilting the screen backward, so that the bottom is closer than the top, can help improve screen visibility providing it doesn't increase screen glare.

- The display attributes, such as brightness and contrast, are adjusted to an easy-to-see brightness and hue setting. The display's brightness and hue may vary depending on the viewing angle.

- The computer screen is placed directly in front of the child and facing them, not angled to the left or right (which encourages neck twisting).

- The eyes are in line with a point on the screen that is 2 to 3 in. below the top of the screen surround. If the screen is above or below this height, your neck will be raised or lowered and the result will be neck pain.

- The screen is at a comfortable viewing distance, which is usually around an arm's length. To check that the screen is properly positioned, you should sit back comfortably in the chair, raise an arm, hold it level at shoulder height and straight in front of you, and your fingers should not quite touch the center of the screen.

- Make sure that text on the screen can easily be read when sitting comfortably. If the text is too small, then either increase magnification factor of the screen (most software programs allow you to zoom in on the screen) or increase the font size, do not move the screen closer to your eyes.

- The child has normally corrected vision. If the child wears glasses, then make sure that they can see the screen without having to adopt an awkward head and neck posture.

- Use a flat-panel, liquid crystal display (LCD) rather than a cathode-ray tube display. An LCD screen presents a stable image to the eyes, which is easier to read, it is less susceptible to screen glare, it is more energy efficient, and it is easier to reposition (see Chapter 3).

Laptop

The goal is to "allow the child to comfortably use a laptop computer in a safe way." This goal can be achieved by ensuring that:

- The child uses a laptop for less than one hour at a time. If the laptop is going to be used for more than one hour per day or as the main computer, it is worthwhile using a mouse or any other external pointing device. Consider obtaining an external keyboard. It is also worth using a laptop stand to raise the screen to viewing height and then docking a separate keyboard and mouse to this. This type of arrangement has been shown to benefit both posture and performance (Berkhout, Hendriksson-Larsen and Bongers, 2004).

- The laptop is used on a work surface at an appropriate height for the child (see Display section) and not on a high surface that will elevate the shoulders and cause shoulder and back pain.

- The laptop has a broad, flat palm rest to intermittently support the child's hands in between bursts of typing on the laptop keyboard.
- The laptop's pointing device is not used exclusively. The central position of the pointing device as is found on almost all laptops may not allow the child to keep their hands and arms in neutral positions while using it for cursor positioning and the position of the input device may result in suboptimal performance (Kelaher, Nay, Lawrence, Lamar and Sommerich, 2001). Taking rest breaks is important!

The risk of problems associated with computer use depends more on the amount of time that one spends keyboarding and mousing without taking a break in one single session than on the total number of keyboarding sessions. Children may not be good at regulating their own computer usage and parents and teachers should be aware of the importance of appropriate intervals and encourage children to learn when to take breaks from computer use.

- Eye Breaks — Looking at a computer screen for a while can cause some changes in how the eyes are working, for example, the rate of blinking will decrease which means that the tear film of the eye is not being refreshed and dirt and debris is not being cleaned from the eye surface as frequently as normal. If the computer screen is incorrectly positioned too high, the upward gaze angle will result in more of the eye surface being exposed to the air. This increase in exposure area combined with a decrease in blink rate will increase the risks of dry, irritated, sore eyes. To minimize these risks, the child should be taught the following regimen — every 20 min they should:
  - Briefly look away from the screen for a minute or two to a more distant scene, preferably something more that 20 ft away, to let the muscles inside the eye relax.
  - Blink the eyes rapidly for a few seconds to refresh the tear film and clear dust form the eye surface.
- Micro-breaks — Most typing and mousing is done intermittently in bursts rather than as continuous movements. Between these bursts of activity children should be taught to rest their hands in a relaxed, flat, straight posture. Working at a computer can be hypnotic, and often children do not realize how long they have been sitting and staring at a screen and how much they have been typing and mousing. It is worthwhile considering the use of ergonomic rest-break software that will run in the background to monitor how much time and how intensely the child has been using the computer, and that provides some visual prompt to take a rest break at appropriate intervals and to perform simple stretching exercises. Following a regimen of taking micro-breaks every 15 min has been shown to

decrease reports of eyestrain and blurred vision, decrease complaints of elbow and arm discomfort, and to produce the highest speed, accuracy, and performance for typical computer tasks (Balci and Aghazadeh, 2003).

- Rest breaks — Every 30 to 60 min children should take a brief rest break when they are allowed to stand up, move around, and do something else other than using the computer. This movement allows the body to rest the muscles used when working at the computer and to exercise different muscles. Moving around promotes better blood circulation, which reduces the accumulation of static muscle fatigue and also promotes alertness.

- Exercise breaks — There are many quick stretching and gentle exercises that children can be taught that can help relieve muscle fatigue. These should be done every 1 to 2 h, depending on the intensity of computer use by the child. In addition to this, encouraging physical fitness will help to reduce injury risks, and promoting ergonomics as part of the school curriculum for physical exercise as well as for computer science will help to reinforce this.

Finally, to obtain the best results these breaks and exercises need to be combined with good workstation setup and good working posture.

Conclusions

As we look to the future, it is highly likely that children will use computers more intensively than they do at present, and consequently ergonomic considerations will become increasingly valuable in ensuring that children do not experience the kinds of visual and musculoskeletal problems that have plagued the adult workforce over the past two decades. To this end, this chapter has briefly summarized our current state of knowledge, as well as providing some concrete guidelines for improving the ergonomic design of computer workstations for children. The chapter has indicated the value of using a variety of ergonomic products that can be found in modern adult office workplaces. However, unlike many private corporations and government organizations, at present many schools and families often do not have the financial resources to provide all children with all of the appropriate furniture and equipment. Although this situation hopefully will change as greater investment is targeted to our children, there is much that can be done by schools and families to improve the ergonomic design of children's computer workstations using minimal resources.

First and foremost, it is important to prioritize the workstation features that most urgently need to be changed based on the needs of those who will be using the workstation and the activities that will be performed. For example, if you know that a computer will primarily be used for word processing, then making sure that the keyboard setup is optimal takes priority. If a computer will be used primarily for graphics design work or for Web surfing, then creating a good mouse/pointing device configuration takes priority.

The single best intervention to make at any computer table or desk is to provide users with a height-adjustable negative-slope keyboard tray that incorporates a height-adjustable mouse platform. However, if the furniture only allows for the desktop use of a keyboard or has a conventional flat or positively sloped articulating tray, then try to position the keyboard as flat as possible, and don't use the feet at the rear of the keyboard. With a lowered, flat surface the keyboard can be tilted downward slightly by placing something underneath the front edge of the keyboard. With desktop keyboard use, providing a broad, flat palm rest that is approximately the same thickness as the front edge of the keyboard for intermittent hand support can help. In the absence of a height and position adjustable mouse tray, at least children can be taught to make sure that the mouse is as close to the side of their body as possible, so that that their upper arm can remain relaxed and their posture can remain as neutral as possible.

In the absence of an adjustable ergonomic chair, using some kind of back cushion and also a removable seat cushion can better accommodate children of various sizes. When children are sitting, if their feet do not reach to the floor, then in the absence of an adjustable footrest it is often possible to provide a makeshift footrest by using a stack of books or a box. A similar approach can be taken to raising the height of the computer screen if this is too low. No doubt readers can generate other creative solutions to suit their particular needs, providing that these follow from the guidelines presented in this chapter. When in doubt concerning any ergonomic guidelines, it is worthwhile to search the Web for additional ergonomics information and to contact ergonomists at universities and colleges.

It is crucial that we heed the warnings of researchers and accept responsibility for ensuring that we do not scar a future generation of computer users by failing to put into practice the ergonomic lessons that we have learned from working with adult computer users.

References

Anshel, J. (1998) *Visual Ergonomics in the Workplace*, Taylor & Francis, London

Armstrong, T., Buckle, B., Fine, L., Hagberg, M., Jonsson, B., Kilbom, A., Kourinka, I., Silverstein, B., Sjogaard, G., and Viikari-Juntura, E. (1993) A conceptual model of work-related neck and upper-limb musculoskeletal disorders. *Scandanavian Journal of Work Environment Health*, 19, 73–84.

Balci, R., Aghazadeh, F. (2003) The effect of work-rest schedules and type of task on the discomfort and performance of VDT users, *Ergonomics*, 46(5), 455–465.

Barrero and Hedge, (2000) School Ergonomics Programs: Guidelines for Parents, http://ergo.human.cornell.edu/MBergo/intro.html Accessed on September 11, 2004.

Berkhout, A.L., Hendriksson-Larsen, K., Bongers, P. (2004) The effect of using a laptop station compared to using a standard laptop pc on the cervical spine torque, perceived strain and productivity, *Applied Ergonomics*, 35(2), 147–152.

Briggs, A., Straker, L., and Greig, A. (2004) Upper quadrant postural changes of school children in response to interaction with different information technologies, *Ergonomics*, 47(7), 790–819.

Buckle, P. and Devereux, J. (1999) *Work-Related Neck And Upper Limb Musculoskeletal Disorders*. Surrey, UK: The Robens Centre for Health Ergonomics, European Institute of Health and Medical Sciences.

Currie, C., Roberts, C., Morgan, A., Smith, R., Settertobulte, W., Samdal, O., and Rasmussen, V.B. (Eds.) (2004) Young people's health in context. Health Behaviour in School-aged Children (HBSC) study: international report from the 2001/2002 survey, Health Policy for Children and Adolescents, No. 4.

DeBell, M. and Chapman, C. (2003) Computer and Internet Use by Children and Adolescents in 2001, NCES 2004–014, U.S. Department of Education, National Center for Education Statistics, Washington, DC. October. (http://nces.ed.gov/pubsearch/pubsinfo.asp?pubid=2004014).

Harris, C., Straker, L. (2000) Survey of physical ergonomics issues associated with school children's use of laptop computers, *International Journal of Industrial Ergonomics*, 26(3), 337–346.

Hedge, A. (1991) Office lighting for VDT work: comparative surveys of reactions to parabolic and lensed indirect systems, In Lovesey, E.J. (ed.) *Contemporary Ergonomics 1991*, Proceedings of the Ergonomics Society Annual Conference, Southampton, England, 16 19 April, (London: Taylor and Francis), 300–305.

Hedge, A., Sims, W.R., and Becker, F.D. (1995) The effects of lensed indirect uplighting and parabolic downlighting on the satisfaction and visual health of office workers, *Ergonomics*, 38(2), 260–280.

Jaschinski, W., Heuer, H., and Kylian, H. (1998) Preferred position of visual displays relative to the eyes: a field study of visual strain and individual differences, *Ergonomics*, 41(7), 1034–1049.

Kelaher, D., Nay, T., Lawrence, B., Lamar, S., and Sommerich, C.M. (2001) An investigation of the effects of touchpad location within a notebook computer, *Applied Ergonomics*, 32(1), 101–110.

Kleiner, A. and Farris, E. (2002) Internet Access in U.S. Public Schools and Classrooms: 1994–2001, U.S. Department of Education, National Center for Education Statistics, NCES 2002-018, Washington, DC, September. (http://nces.ed.gov/pubsearch/pubsinfo.asp?pubid=2002018).

Kumar, S. (2001) Theories of musculoskeletal injury causation, *Ergonomics*, 44(1), 17–47.

Laeser, K.L., Maxwell, L.E. and Hedge, A. (1998) The effects of computer workstation design on student posture, *Journal of Research on Computing in Education*, 31(2), 173–188.

Marumoto, T., Sotoyama, M., Villanueva, M.B.G., Jonai, H., Yamada, H., Kanai, A., and Saito, S. (1996) Relationship between sitting posture and eye accommodation of young students, *Proceedings of the 4th Pan Pacific Conference on Occupational Ergonomics*, Taipei, Taiwan, November 11–13, 1996. Ergonomics Society of Taiwan, Hsinchu, Taiwan, 208–211.

Marumoto, T., Sotoyama, M., Villanueva, M.B.G., Jonai, H., Yamada, H., Kanai, A., and Saito, S. (1999) Significant correlation between school myopia and postural parameters of students while studying, *International Journal of Industrial Ergonomics*, 23(1–2), 33–39.

McAtamney, L. and Corlett, E.N. (1993) RULA: a survey method for the investigation of work-related upper limb disorders, *Applied Ergonomics*, 24, 91–99.

NRC-IOM (2001) Musculoskeletal Disorders And The Workplace: Low Back and Upper Extremities, Panel on Musculoskeletal Disorders and the Workplace, Commission on Behavioral and Social Sciences and Education, National Research Council and Institute of Medicine, National Academy Press, Washington, D.C.

Oates, S., Evans, G., and Hedge, A. (1998) A preliminary ergonomic and postural assessment of computer work settings in American elementary schools, *Computers in the Schools*, 14, 3/4, 55–63.

Rideout, V. J., Vandewater, E. A., and Wartella, E. A. (2003) Zero to six: Electronic media in the lives of infants, toddlers and preschoolers, A Kaiser Family Foundation Report (http://www.kff.org/entmedia/3378.cfm)

Saito, S., Piccoli, B., Smith, M.J., Sotoyama, M., Sweitzer, G., Villanueva, M.B.G., and Yoshitake, R. (2000) Ergonomic guidelines for using notebook personal computers, *Industrial Health*, 38(4), 421–434. http://www.niih.go.jp/jp/indu_hel/2000/pdf/IH38_55.pdf.

Straker L. (2001) Are children at more risk of developing musculoskeletal disorders from working with computers or with paper? *Advances in Occupational Ergonomics and Safety*, Amsterdam: IOS Press, July, 344–353.

Straker, L., Harris, C., and Zandvliet, D. (2000) Scarring a generation of school children through poor introduction of information technology in schools. *Ergonomics for the New Millennium*, Proceedings of the XIVth Triennial Congress of the International Ergonomics Association and the 44th Annual Meeting of the Human Factors and Ergonomics Society, San Diego, CA, July 29-August 4, 2000. Human Factors and Ergonomics Society, Santa Monica, CA, Volume 6, 300–303.

Straker, L. Briggs, A., and Grieg, A. (2002) The effect of individually adjusted workstations on upper quadrant posture and muscle activity in school children, *WORK: A Journal of Prevention, Assessment, and Rehabilitation*, 18, 239–248.

Vryzas, K., Tsitouridou, M. (2002) The home computer in children's everyday life: the case of Greece, *Journal of Educational Media*, 27(1-2), 9–17.

10

General Eye Care Tips

Jeffrey Anshel

CONTENTS

Introduction

This chapter is intended to be a sort of catch-all to bring together some peripheral ideas and concerns regarding computer use. We will examine such ideas as nutrition, aging, contact lenses, exercises, and more. It may appear on the surface that some of these ideas have nothing to do with computer use, but these are areas that can affect your ability to use a computer display comfortably. These concepts can be considered an aspect of holistic health care where it is advantageous to consider the whole person or process.

Stress and Vision

Stress is something we live with every day. It has become an integral part of our workdays, as well as other aspects of our lives. It has positive and negative effects on our biological system, many of which are beyond the scope of this discussion. However, we will touch on the subject to emphasize the importance of stress reduction in maintaining good vision and good working habits.

We normally associate stress with muscle tension. While the two are actually different processes, it has become commonplace to accept the notion that stress usually leads to increased (excessive) muscle tension. There are many areas of our bodies where this muscle tension tends to manifest. Since this is a discussion of the visual system, the focus will be limited to the visual stress associated with computer work.

Stress can easily affect vision. Measuring how this occurs is not a routine clinical process since stress is often simply a subjective symptom. Yet the eye and visual system are directly connected to the brain, so measuring brain waves can be an indication of visual stress. The electroencephalogram (EEG) has been used to measure the brain waves of people experiencing visual stress (Pierce, 1966). It was found that there are changes in other bodily functions, including heartbeat, respiration, and blood vessel size, as well as an overflow to other nonvisual brain areas that can occur with a visually demanding task. The earliest EEG studies in the 1920s confirmed that visual input affected brain-wave patterns. Scientists have established not only that the EEG pattern could be changed by repetitive visual stimulation at a known frequency, but also that the brain would quickly respond by falling into that same frequency. This process is employed in practice during vision therapy to elicit a relaxation response by a patient. The frequency of stimulation is in the range of 8 to 12 Hz, which approximates the alpha rhythm, or relaxed state of the brain. One might speculate what effects, negative or otherwise, might be elicited by viewing a 75 Hz flashing image (a CRT display screen) during the course of an 8-hour workday. While there are no reports of any negative flicker effects of display viewing, we know that various flicker frequencies can cause different reactions.

The reaction to visual stress can take many forms. One reaction is to avoid doing the stressful task. Another is to do the work but approach it with reduced comprehension while experiencing physical discomfort. A third is to physically adapt to the stressful situation. This third adaptation could include the development of myopia or the suppression of one eye's image. Figure 10.1 shows the various adaptations to visual stress one might make.

Billette and Piche (1987) and Bergman (1980), among others, have noted a significant relationship between stress and job function. Often it is the job design and not the worker that is the cause of stress. Some jobs are inherently more stressful than others. For example, an air traffic controller, whose responsibility for the safety of thousands of people on a daily basis must be considered differently from that of a mail clerk, who may occasionally glance at a display screen. In general, the more controlled, timed, repetitive, and socially isolated the job, the more stressful it tends to be. Jobs that provide more latitude for the worker to control the job pace and design of the work are the easiest to deal with.

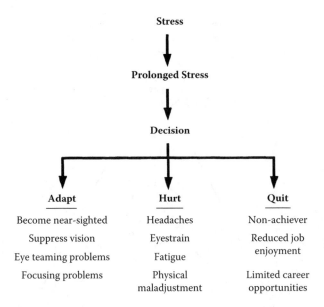

FIGURE 10.1
Our eyes will adapt to stress in a variety of ways (after Godnig, 1990).

In addition to the organization of the work, other environmental factors affect the stress level of the worker. Factors leading to job stress include poor lighting, excessive noise levels, unhealthy air quality, inadequate workspace, and poorly designed furniture and workstations.

So we can now see that there are many factors that affect stress of computer users. Figure 10.2 illustrates some of the main areas that need to be addressed.

Eye Health Concerns

Video displays, like all electrical devices, give off a small amount of electro-magnetic radiation. This radiation is energy that moves through space at various frequencies. The radiation spectrum is divided between high-frequency ionizing radiation, and lower-frequency nonionizing radiation (Figure 10.3). X-radiation, such as that used for medical purposes, is a type of ionizing radiation while sunlight consists of several types of nonionizing radiation including visible light, ultraviolet, and infrared.

Computer displays produce several types of radiation, including x-radiation, infrared (heat), visible light, radio frequency, ultraviolet and others. The cathode ray tube functions by using a stream of electrons that energizes the phosphors to cause illumination. Side products of that process include several types of optical radiation including ultraviolet, visible and infrared

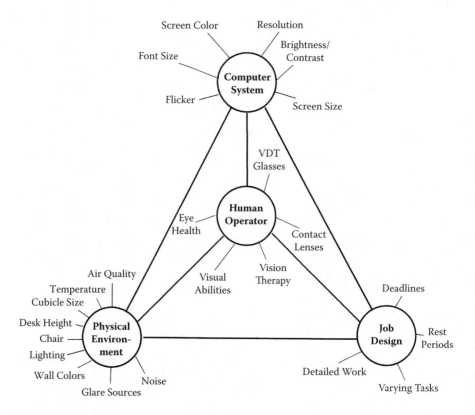

FIGURE 10.2
Factors affecting computer viewing stress (after Godnig, 1990).

radiation. The electrical circuitry, including the transformer produces infrared and various types of radio frequency radiation.

It is very difficult to determine what subtle effects, if any, low-frequency fields may have on living tissue over long periods. It is known that the body's cells have their own electric fields, and some laboratory studies have shown that these internal fields can be disrupted by exposure to even low-energy electromagnetic fields (EMF). Some scientists hypothesize that subsequent cell changes — notably in cell membranes, genetic material, immune function, and hormonal and enzyme activity — may lead to increased cancer risk. It is, however, difficult to extrapolate from test-tube studies to human beings living in the real world.

The stream of electrons by which computers display images on screen generates fields in the very-low frequency (VLF) and extremely low frequency (ELF) range, which pass right through the machine's case. It's the magnetic fields that scientists are most concerned about and that are hardest to shield. Various appliances produce similar energy fields, but the distinctive type from a computer display is emitted in sharp bursts, which may have a greater effect on tissue.

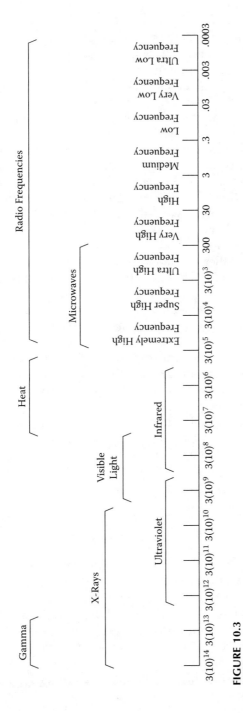

FIGURE 10.3
The electromagnetic spectrum.

Concern about display radiation began in the early 1970s when reports appeared about computer operators having high rates of headaches, miscarriages, cataracts, and other health problems. There have been various reports of findings for and against caution, but thus far no conclusive evidence has shown that there are any significant long-term effects from computer use. The National Institutes of Health concluded that any effects of the display itself did not cause the apparent miscarriage rate for computer users. The reports of computer users having a higher than normal incidence of cataracts has also been disputed as a side effect of the many users who are elderly, when cataract formation is more common. No substantiated negative health effect on the eye has been caused specifically from computer use.

On the side of caution, however, it is probably prudent to minimize the risk of exposure, especially if you are a full-time user on a video display. Electromagnetic radiation falls off rapidly with distance from the source. Try to maintain at least a 24-in. working distance from the screen and also be sure that there are no other monitors in your immediate vicinity. It has been shown that more radiation comes from the back or sides of the monitor than through the screen. There has been no evidence that warrants ultraviolet protection in glasses that are worn for computer use. It has been shown that the amount of ultraviolet light emanating from the screen is minimal and no cause for concern. When shopping for a monitor, make sure it complies with the Swedish standards, which most new monitors do. Also, do not succumb to anti-glare screen ads that tout that they block radiation. Although these may block low-frequency electric fields, they do not block magnetic fields, which are a greater concern.

The newer LCD displays should offer a sense of relief to computer users since they produce only a fraction of the amount of ELF radiation of a traditional CRT display. More information regarding visual display technology is presented in Chapter 3.

Aging Factors

The Bureau of Labor Statistics estimates that by 2008, the age group 55 years and older will grow by 14 million, as compared with 1998. This age group will make up 20% of the work force by 2012. It would be highly unlikely to assume that these older workers will be doing manual labor type of work. Instead, the trend for the older worker is to do some type of desk work that involves the use of a computer. Let's examine the various considerations that older workers must address in their computer-viewing environments.

The most significant condition facing the vision of the older worker is presbyopia. As you learned in Chapter 2, presbyopia is the loss of accommodation with age, which usually becomes apparent after the age of 40. The presbyopic person must hold their reading material at a farther distance if they hope to see it clearly. One advantage of using a computer in the workplace is that it is most often (as it should be) placed farther away from the eye than is printed reading material. For the pre-presbyopic (younger than 40 years old) viewer who does not use reading glasses, this could delay the symptoms of presbyopia. However, once reading glasses are prescribed to compensate for the loss of accommodation, caution must be taken to ensure that the entire viewing area is available.

Since a reading distance of 16 in. is the standard testing range for eye exams, this is the area of clear near viewing obtained through reading glasses. If a display screen is set at 28 in., for example, it may not be clear through the glasses. If a presbyopic person uses bifocals, the reading portion is normally situated in the lower portion of the lens to allow for clear reading in a lowered-eye position. The display screen is most often situated in a higher visual field position, thereby requiring a bifocal wearer to tilt the head up in order to read through the bifocal lens to see the screen. This can (and usually does) create a problem with neck and shoulder pain.

Even the use of the progressive addition lens (PAL), often referred to as the no-line bifocal, is not usually acceptable for prolonged computer viewing. The intermediate range segment of the lens is often too narrow to provide extended viewing comfort. Using computer glasses, with or without lines, which are designed specifically for the working distance and viewing angle of the VDT screen, will usually resolve most problems.

Lighting in the workplace can also become a significant factor with the aging of the workforce. A 60-year-old worker needs many times more light than a 20 year old. If the workplace has younger and older workers in the same area, a proper balance of light should be available to please both age groups. Task lighting usually provides the best resolution to this problem. Lighting is discussed more fully in Chapter 5.

Dry eyes are a very common condition in the elderly population, especially for women. It appears that changes in hormone levels can adversely affect the tear layer formation, leading to a dry-eye condition. While it is difficult to make specific recommendations as to what to do for dry eyes without a full eye examination, artificial tears (not eye whiteners) and vitamins are a few remedies that have shown some success. The traditional artificial tear has been a temporary measure and is relatively unsuccessful in reducing the symptoms of dry eyes. Newer drops offer better effectiveness. A vitamin option is discussed in a subsequent section.

Another area of concern for the aging computer user is a condition known as age-related macular degeneration (AMD). As you'll recall from Chapter 2, the macula is the central part of the retina that is responsible for our sharpest vision (20/20). Because the blood supply to that area is so minimal, the few blood vessels that supply that area have a tendency to break down after many years. This causes a degeneration of the retinal cells in that area. While it doesn't lead to complete blindness, the main result is a loss of clear vision at the central point of vision.

For computer users, this means that the smaller text of a typical document might be obscured. One way to work around this is to enlarge the letters so that they strike the retina on an area around the damaged central area. While that serves to make reading slower, it will allow the individual to be productive.

A fifth area of concern in the aging worker is the formation of cataracts. The crystalline lens within the eye (that is responsible for accommodation) can become cloudy with age. By definition, any cloudiness in the lens is called a cataract. However, slight clouding and yellowing of the lens is considered normal for the aging person. If the cloudiness becomes excessive, or clouds the central seeing part of the lens, then the cataract will inhibit light through the lens. This will block the individual's vision.

Cataract surgery is the most common surgery performed in the U.S. annually. Fortunately, newer techniques and replacement lenses are now available so that the patient can see very clearly following the procedure. There is no reason for the patient to wait until the cataract "ripens," as was once the case. If the employee is diagnosed with a cataract, then the outpatient procedure can be done with likely no complications. A full evaluation by the surgeon can determine whether the procedure is appropriate.

Computers and Contacts

We briefly touched on the subject of contact lenses previously while discussing eye exams and glasses (Chapter 7). In addition, there are some considerations that should be noted for the computer worker who wears contact lenses during the workday.

It has already been pointed out that dry eye is one of the significant symptoms of computer vision syndrome. This condition can be exacerbated greatly by the use of contact lenses. Since the contact lens is essentially a piece of plastic floating on the tear layer of the eye, it can be susceptible to dry environmental conditions. If the lens wearer has a marginally dry eye condition, wears contact lenses, and uses a computer regularly, then a dry eye feeling is likely to manifest during or after computer use. The regular use of an artificial tear substitute eye drop has traditionally been recommended to relieve this symptom. Some better options to relieve this condition are listed in a subsequent section.

Often the room in which the display is used is an arid environment due to the requirements of the computer's CPU. The CPU must not be exposed to a high-humidity environment, so the air in these rooms can be especially dry. This, again, can lead to noticeable symptoms of dry eyes while using contact lenses. The display screen itself has an electromagnetic charge, and therefore attracts dust. These dust particles can often lodge under a contact lens causing discomfort. Lens removal and rewetting is a simple solution to this problem.

For visual correction, contact lenses are routinely prescribed to correct distance vision problems. Wiggins et al. (1992) found that the incomplete correction of astigmatism in contact lens wearers using display screens created symptoms of visual stress. If this distance prescription is adequate for near/intermediate use as well, no problems should be noted. However, if the near/intermediate vision correction is different than that for distance, the contact lens wearer may experience other symptoms of computer vision syndrome. It is possible to wear computer glasses in addition to the contact lenses.

Vitamins and VDTs

This section is not intended to offer specific remedies to have your display look better or live longer by giving it a specific vitamin regimen. However, it is intended to offer you some suggestions that you might want to incorporate into your own diet that might relieve some symptoms that may be experienced while viewing your display screen.

Let's take yet another look at the dry eye condition. There are two causes for dry eyes: 1) not enough tears (quantity); or 2) rapidly evaporating tears (quality). It is relatively rare for a dry eye condition to be caused by a decreased quantity of tears. Many successful contact lens patients have a very low volume of tears. The glands within the lining of the eye maintain the normal tear volume. But the tears you experience while crying are produced by a gland in the upper corner of the bony orbit, just behind your eyebrow. The quality of the tears, which maintains their integrity so they do not evaporate too quickly, is the more important concern. This quality of tear is dependent on a fatty layer that covers the watery layer of tears. If this fatty layer is deficient, it will break up quickly, allowing the water tear layer to evaporate too quickly and leading to a dry eye symptom. One of the most important factors in maintaining this fatty layer is vitamin A (or beta-carotene). Patel, et al. (1991) showed that vitamin A is essential in maintaining the stability of the tear film on the eye. Omega-3 and omega-6 fatty acids, flaxseed oil, borage oil, and selenium are just a few other nutrients that have been shown to be effective in maintaining a good quality tear film.

Vitamin A is just one of the group of nutrients known as antioxidants. This group of vitamins and minerals is useful in reducing the effect of oxygen free radicals on living tissue. The foundation of this research is beyond the scope of this book but there are some key issues that should be kept in mind. The group of antioxidants includes vitamin A (beta carotene), vitamin C, vitamin E, selenium, inositol, panthothene, and zinc. These have been shown to be effective in reducing the severity of cataract formation and the condition of age-related macular degeneration. More research is being conducted as of this writing but it looks very promising that vitamin and mineral supplements can enhance our resistance to certain types of diseases and disorders.

General Body Exercises

Throughout this text we have maintained the notion that the eyes are an integral part of the body and must be treated in much the same way — with attention and care. Since the "eyes lead the body," it only makes sense that good body exercises will help you to maintain good posture at the workstation. Here are some general body exercises that are easy to do and very effective (Figure 10.4). A word of caution: if you have any pre-existing condition that might be aggravated by doing these exercises, please consult with your health care provider prior to attempting them.

A. Pectoral stretch: Do this when you find yourself slouching. Clasp your hands behind your head. Tuck in your chin, press the back of your head into your hands, and push your elbows as far back as you can. Hold for 3 seconds, then relax and repeat 5 times.

B. Disk reliever: Do this to reverse the effects of repetitive or sustained bending. Place your hands in the hollow of your back. While focusing your eyes straight ahead, bend backward over your hands without bending your knees, then immediately straighten up.

C. Pelvic tilt: Do this to reverse the effects of standing with "sway back." Begin by standing with your back to the wall. Tighten your stomach muscles to flatten your back. Hold for several seconds. Once you've mastered the exercise, do it sitting or standing.

D. Wrist/finger: Hold one hand with fingers upward. Gently push fingers and wrist back with the other hand. Hold for 3 sec. Repeat 5 times for each hand.

E. Thumb: Hold one hand with fingers upward. Gently pull back the thumb with the fingers of the other hand. Hold for 3 sec. Repeat 5 times for each hand.

F. Whole hand: Spread the fingers of both hands apart and back while keeping your wrists straight. Hold for 3 sec. Repeat this exercise 5 times for each hand.

G. Head roll: Relax your shoulders and pull your head forward as far as it will go. Hold for just two seconds. Then slowly rotate your head along your shoulders until it is all the way back. Continue rolling around to the other side until you return to your original position. Roll you head in one direction three cycles, then reverse

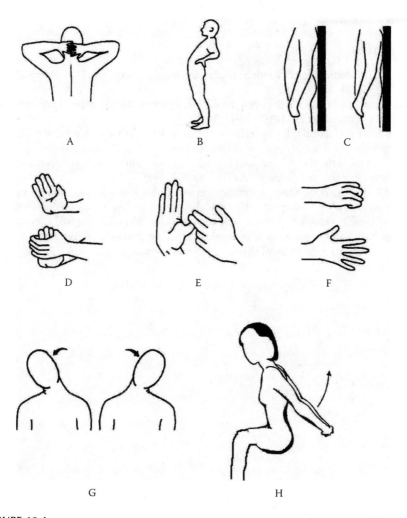

FIGURE 10.4
Try these easy exercises to get your blood flowing properly and keep your energy while using your computer.

the direction for another three cycles. Feel the upper shoulder muscles relax. Do these slowly and feel the stretch in the neck muscles.

H. Shoulder squeeze: Another excellent stretch for slouchers. Lace your fingers behind your back with the palms facing in. Slowly raise and straighten your arms. Hold for 5 to 10 sec. Repeat 5 to 10 times.

While doing all of these exercises, it is important to remember to maintain a full and smooth breathing pace. Full breaths allow for further relaxation of the muscles being stretched. They also allow for increased blood circulation, which will improve your alertness and mental activity.

References

Bergman, T. Health effects of video display terminals, *Occup. Health & Safety*, (Nov/ Dec) 24-28, 53-55; 1980.

Billete, A. and Piche, J. Health problems of data entry clerks and related job stressors, *J. of Occup. Med.*, 29 (12), 942-948, 1987.

Godnig, E. and Hacunda, J. *Computers and Visual Stress*. Abacus, Grand Rapids, MI, 1991.

Patel, S., et al. Effect of visual display unit use on blink rate and tear stability, *Optometry & Vision Science*, 68 (11), 888-892, 1991.

Pierce, J.R. Research on the relationship between near point lenses, human performance, and physiological activity of the body, Optometric Extension Program Courses, Research Reports and Special Articles, 39 (1-12), 1966-67.

Wiggins, N.P. and Daum, K.M. Effects of residual astigmatism in contact lens wear on visual discomfort in VDT use, *J. American Optom. Assn.*, 63(3), 177-181, 1992.

11

Economics of Visual Ergonomics

Maurice Oxenburgh and Pepe Marlow

CONTENTS

Financial Modeling

When it comes to arguing for funds to be expended, to just present the cost of a project does not reflect its value to the enterprise. If several projects are competing for funding then, in financial terms, the project that provides the greatest value should be funded first. Financial modeling can be used to calculate the value of a future project, incorporating both its costs and expected benefits quantitatively.

In the engineering field it is usual for engineers to prepare a cost-benefit analysis to support their project, with productivity data selected and costed and the benefits estimated on the basis of custom and practice. In contrast, ergonomists are often cautious about making predictions about the benefits of a project, particularly predictions about reduced injury occurrences.

We suggest ergonomists follow the lead of engineers in making use of cost-benefit analysis tools. Engineers have developed cost-benefit models that suit the questions they want to answer such as: "Should we buy that new machine or should we continue to maintain the old one?" Engineers are also comfortable with the need to make estimates on the basis of their experience.

In a cost-benefit analysis, one uses historical data and experience to make predictions about the future and hence can only estimate costs and benefits. In presenting an analysis, it is important to specify the assumptions on which the calculations have been based and, in this way, the limitations of the analysis will be clearly understood.

Used judiciously, cost-benefit analysis can be a powerful tool for presenting your argument for funding any ergonomics project. Cost-benefit analysis enables benefits of an ergonomics intervention for that enterprise to be quantified, presenting the value of the intervention to the enterprise's decision makers. Think of cost-benefit analysis as simply a tool to assist in asserting your point of view about the need for ergonomics interventions.

Cost-benefit analysis is an economic model and to use it effectively in situations where your proposal is competing for funds against other projects, it is necessary to understand at least some of the economics behind it.

Cost-Benefit Analysis

Cost-Benefit Analysis Assumptions

A cost-benefit analysis assumes that the present work situation is not optimal and that changes (an intervention) may be made to improve worker productivity and other cost factors, including injury and absence costs. To do this, the cost-benefit analysis assesses a workplace at a particular point in time, for example now, and compares it with future or alternative situations, termed the test cases.

In the particular cost-benefit analysis model presented in this chapter, the major determinate is of the workers who produce the goods or services and not of the goods or services themselves. By contrast, most analyses take as their starting point the equipment and manufacturing processes or service, making them unsuitable to measure the people side. When an enterprise is deciding where to spend its money, all approaches (people, goods, or services) need to be integrated but, for the purposes of this chapter, we will concentrate on the people side.

Certain cost data need to be gathered for a cost-benefit analysis and, if costs are not accurately known, then estimates are required. The data required include:

- The important and critical data relating to employment costs — the costs of the current situation
- The costs for implementing the intervention in the workplace
- The benefits due to the intervention

Costs of the Current Situation

In costing the current situation, some of the employment data required are straightforward and usually easy to obtain. These include the direct labor costs of hours worked, wages, social costs, training, absenteeism, etc., and, where appropriate, may also include a portion of the organizational costs of supervision, management, and head office costs.

Other data may be less easy to obtain but, in our experience, give the greatest return on ergonomics investment. These include:

- Productivity (gross output and quality)
- Labor turnover
- Error and warranty costs
- Equipment and material costs (equipment failures, waste, errors, etc.)

Where these costs are not known one can include an estimate for costs that are expected to change, for better or worse, due to the intervention.

Costing the Intervention

Where costs for the intervention may vary it would be useful to prepare more than one test case. Suggested bases for preparing test cases are:

- The minimum expected cost and maximum expected cost
- The cost for each stage in a staged project
- The break-even point, that is the maximum cost that would equal the benefits gained from the project

Costing the Benefits

The process of making estimates about benefits are little different from the warehouse manager who wants a new forklift truck, the call center manager who wants new computer software, or the hotel manager who requires more cleaning staff. The cost of the forklift truck may be known but the benefits are only assumptions; will the forklift truck reduce loading time and goods damage? By a similar argument, will the new software bring in more telephone customers? Will the extra staff increase the standard, and the guest fees, of the hotel? Determining the future can only be based on the best guesses, even when based on experience.

Cost-Benefit Analysis Data Checklist

Most ergonomists will be familiar with checklists to assist in determining work tasks, work organization, or workstations. Collecting data for a cost-benefit analysis model can act as a checklist to identify economic parameters with which the ergonomist will be less familiar.

One essential feature of any checklist must be the *relevance* of the questions it poses. In our experience finding the data is not usually too difficult; asking the *relevant* questions is the crux of the matter. A cost-benefit analysis model must direct the user to the relevant questions but still allow the user to determine the appropriateness of the individual questions.

A Cost-Benefit Analysis Model, the Productivity Assessment Tool

Unfortunately, there is a dearth of generic cost-benefit analysis models specifically directed to occupational ergonomics, health, and safety. Several analyses have been published (for example, see *Applied Ergonomics*, 2003), but they are usually specific to a particular case and not developed as a generic model.

In this chapter, we will describe one generic cost-benefit analysis model (the Productivity Assessment Tool) developed for use by ergonomists and other occupational health and safety practitioners.

A basic software version of the Productivity Assessment Tool has been published in Oxenburgh et al., (2004), which allows one employee or employee group and one test case for comparison with the initial or current situation. The model is equally applicable for service or manufacturing industries.

The full version of the Productivity Assessment Tool (ProductAbility, 2004) allows the user to include the costs for up to five individual employees or employee groups in the selected workplace. This flexibility can accommodate differences in working hours, pay rates, overtime, absenteeism, and productivity. With the reduction in full-time or permanent employment and the concomitant rise in precarious or casual employment (Bohle and Quinlan, 2000), such employment variations are common.

In addition, in the full version of the software the current or unimproved state of the workplace (the initial case) can be compared with up to four possible interventions (the test cases). The advantage is that one can propose several possible solutions to any problem and directly compare their economic effectiveness. Needless to say, ergonomists must use their core skills to judge that these test cases will be comparable in terms of injury prevention, or other worker benefits, before putting them forward for funding supported by a cost-benefit analysis.

Case Studies

Safety Signs and Conspicuity

This is a case study, derived from the original work of Adams and Montague (1994), which we are using to illustrate the essential points in a cost-benefit analysis.

In the Australian outback, the hamlets and towns are far apart and the task of maintaining the railway tracks goes to small gangs of men working in isolation, far from these population centers.

The injury rate among the gangers was not acceptable, but neither were the means of injury prevention. In a gang of, for example, eight men, four of the men would be designated as flagmen. The role of the four flagmen was to warn the approaching trains of the hazard of men working on the track. Two men were positioned on either side of the track-work some distance away; on the approach of a train, the flagmen would hold a flag horizontally at the side of the track.

Although the train driver would be informed of the approximate whereabouts of the track work at the start of the shift this may have been some hours previous and perhaps many hundreds of kilometers away. It was not unknown for a driver to miss these warning flags, with unfortunate consequences.

In addition to the safety factors, there were productivity factors. In the case of an eight-man gang, only four would be involved in actual track maintenance with the other four as flagmen. The cost factor of having one half of a team not engaged in track maintenance was not good economics.

Clearly a better method was needed to warn train drivers that they were approaching a track gang both for safety reasons and improved productivity.

The drivers, unions, and the railways authority all had considerable input into the discussions for a safer and more productive signaling system and it was agreed that large sign boards could substitute for the flag men. They had to be big enough to be seen although small enough to be manageable and the agreed size was 400 mm × 1200 mm (about 16 × 48 in.) with three boards to be placed on either side of the track gang. One board was to be at 2.5 km (about 1.5 miles) and another at 2 km (about 1 mile) from the track work and another at 500 m (about 550 yards) from the track work.

There were disagreements regarding the suitability and visibility of the various suggestions for the signboards. As no agreement was forthcoming, and it was clearly the crucial issue, it was agreed that the solution was to employ independent consultants to prepare and test signboards.

Three consultants were employed, including a designer and a psychologist, and they tested their designs on 19 railway workers.

The test system the consultants devised involved a photograph of a country railway line with the test signboards, scaled to the apparent size of this country scene, mounted on the photograph. The test personnel then walked toward the photograph, starting from a distance of 25 m, and had to state (1) when they could first see a sign (conspicuity), and then (2) when they could discriminate which sign it was — the 2.5-km, 2-km or 500-m sign.

Clearly, the further away they could see and determine the sign, the more conspicuous, selective, and safe the sign was. By this testing system, a suitable design was selected.

The costs for the test system were the wages and time of the research workers (designers and psychologist), the cost of meetings between the consultants and the clients (the senior railway authority personnel) and the cost of participation of the test subjects (the railway workers).

The cost for the test procedure, see Table 11.1, was about $25,000 and this can be assumed to be the intervention cost. In actual fact, one should add the cost of the signs but this was comparatively minor and is ignored in this example.

Table 11.2 shows the cost-benefit analysis. It examines the cost benefit for two different sizes of track gangs, one with eight men (rows 1 and 2) and one with 12 men (rows 3 and 4). In each case, four men were initially employed as flagmen and this is shown in rows 1 and 3 respectively. The wage costs of $31 per man, per hour included provision for holidays and supervision but did not include illness absence costs or administrative costs.

TABLE 11.1

Cost of the Intervention

Category and Number of Persons	Total Hours	Wages or Consultant Cost per Hour	Net Amount in $
3 consultants	104	$200 per hour	20,800
1 research assistant	24	$60 per hour	1,440
19 subjects	19	$31 per hour	589
Meetings with railway authority managers, union officials	25	$100 per hour	2,500
Total wage, salary, and consultant costs			25,329

TABLE 11.2
Cost-Benefit Analysis of the Test System

Row Number	Number in a Gang	Wages/hr ($)	Number of Flagmen	Number Working on Track Maintenance	Cost/Day ($)	Total Wage Costs for Track Gang ($/Year)	Loss of Productivity due to Flag Men ($/Year)	Savings ($/Year)	Pay-back Period[a] (Weeks)
1 flag men	8	31	4	4	1,984	466,000	233,000		
2 sign posts	8	31	0	8	1,984	466,000	0	233,000	5
3 flag men	12	31	4	8	2,976	699,000	233,000		
4 sign posts	12	31	0	12	2,976	699,000	0	233,000	5

[a] Intervention cost was $25,329.

Rows 2 and 4 show the economic impact of the intervention when the safety signs were introduced to replace the flagmen. The savings, due to the introduction of the safety signs, was $233,000 per year for each gang.

The payback period was only five weeks regardless of whether the gangs consisted of 8 or 12 men. This is because the intervention cost is small relative to the productivity gained by freeing up 4 men to perform maintenance work. In actual fact the payback period is less than this as the testing costs should be distributed across all the track maintenance gangs: for example, if there are 10 gangs, then only 10% of the intervention costs should be included in the cost-benefit analysis for each gang.

Welders' Eye Safety

Although personal protective equipment is a last resort for safety, in some cases it is an essential element. In the words of the ILO (International Labor Office, 1997):

> First and foremost, the selection and proper use of protective clothing should be based on an assessment of the hazards involved in the task for which the protection is required. In light of the assessment, an accurate definition of the performance requirements and the ergonomic constraints of the job can be determined. Finally, a selection that balances worker protection, ease of use, and cost can be made.

Automatic darkening welding helmets are a case in point. They are very expensive and do not protect the eyes any better than the conventional helmets. Why spend more?

The answer to this question lies in economics and is an example of the full use of cost-benefit analysis.

This case study concerns a small company manufacturing metal beds, bed heads, and accessories (for full details, see Oxenburgh et al., 2004). It is a highly competitive industry and, although this company survives in a market where most of its competitors have gone out of business, it is now facing stiff import competition. High productivity is essential if it is to stay in business.

Of the 16 full-time employees, only three are welders. The other employees work on painting, assembly, warehousing, and delivery.

A considerable number of spot welds are required in the fabrication of the bed heads and other metal furniture. Due to the large variety of bed head designs and sizes, the output varies considerably on a day-by-day basis. However, there are usually 10 welds required per bed head and, as the bed head has to be turned around to weld the other side, it means that each bed head requires 20 separate applications of the welding torch. In one hour, a welder would weld about 12 bed heads so that the welding torch is applied to 240 separate welding spots per welder, per hour.

Normally, the welder would have to raise his conventional helmet for each weld but the use of the automatic darkening welding helmet has enabled the welder to weld a whole side of the bed head (10 welds) without having to raise his helmet.

In many ways, this is an exceptional case of spot welding as the welders only do spot welds and, except for setting up their jobs in the jigs, have no other tasks. It can be conservatively estimated that if the welders did not have the automatic darkening welding helmets and were only supplied with conventional welding helmets, then one extra welder would be needed.

Table 11.3 shows the cost-benefit analysis for the purchase of automatic darkening welding helmets. The number of welders would have been four if the conventional helmet had been worn (second column) whereas only three welders, using automatic darkening welding helmets (third column), are needed.

A payback period of three weeks can leave one in no doubt as to the cost advantages of using this particular piece of eye protection equipment and shows the advantages of exploring the *cost effectiveness* of personal protective equipment rather than only looking at the purchase price.

TABLE 11.3

Cost Benefit Analysis for Welders — Metal Bed Head Manufacture

	Conventional Helmet	Automatic Darkening Helmet
Employment Costs		
Number of welders	4	3
Paid time per worker (40 hour week); hour/year	2,080	2,080
Time paid but not worked (vacation, illness, etc.); hour/year	256	256
Productive time (actual time worked); hour/year	1,824	1,824
Wage paid directly to each welder; $/hour	17.50	17.50
Employment cost (wages plus overheads; workers compensation, pension, and supervisory costs); $/hour	23.88	23.88
Productive employment cost (employment cost per productive hour); $/hour	27.24	27.24
Fixed employment cost for all the welders; $/year	198,720	149,040
Intervention costs (purchase of three automatic darkening helmets); $	—	2,800
Savings (assumed to occur in one year); $/year	—	48,320
Payback period;[a] weeks	—	3

[a] The payback period is the time period (wage savings) to pay for purchase of the automatic darkening welding helmets.

Conclusion

In this chapter the authors have shown that economics, in the form of cost benefit analysis, may play a part in all manner of ergonomics interventions, including visual ergonomics. That is *not* to say that, when considering an ergonomics intervention, one should only include financial considerations in the process; the true use of economics is to assist in improving the human condition — it is not an end in itself.

In a nutshell, one uses the concept of the cost benefit of a proposed ergonomics intervention in order to *compete* for limited resources. Of course other means are available for this competition (e.g., legal requirements, moral issues) and can be used with or without financial considerations. However, in our experience, financial considerations, more often than not, determine which solutions are implemented.

References

Adams A. S. and Montague M., 1994. Testing warning signs: conspicuity and discrimination. *Information Design Journal*, 7(3), 203–210.

Applied Ergonomics (vol. 34 [5] September 2003). A Special Issue devoted to cost effectiveness.

Bohle P. and Quinlan M., 2000. *Managing Occupational Health and Safety.* 2nd edition (Melbourne: Macmillan).

International Labor Office, 1997. From the *Encyclopaedia of Occupational Health and Safety*, 4th Edition, (Geneva).

Oxenburgh M., Marlow P., and Oxenburgh, A., 2004. *Increasing Productivity and Profit through Health & Safety: The Financial Returns from a Safe Working Environment*, 2nd edition. CRC Press, Boca Raton, FL.

ProductAbility, 2004. Software for the Productivity Assessment Tool (Copyright; Oxenburgh, M. and Matchbox Software Ltd., U.K. See www.productability.co.uk).

Appendix A

Computer Workplace Questionnaire

Work Practices:

1. Number of hours per workday of computer viewing _____
2. How long have you worked at a computer job? _____
3. Type of work habits: (circle one)
   a. Intermittent — periods of less than 1 hour
   b. Intermittent — periods of more than 1 hour
   c. Constant — informal breaks, as required
   d. Constant — regular breaks
   e. Constant— no breaks, other than meals
4. How often do you clean your display screen? _____

Environment:

Lighting in the work area: (check all that apply)
Fluorescent overhead only _____
Incandescent overhead only _____
Fluorescent and incandescent overhead _____
Fluorescent overhead and incandescent direct _____
Window light _____ In front? Behind? To the side?
Window light control: Curtains? Blinds? Vertical/Horizontal?
Desk Lamp/Task Light _____
How would you rate the brightness of the room?
   Very bright / Medium / Dim

Display Screen:

What color are the letters on your screen? _____
What color is the background of your screen? _____

Viewing distance from your eye to display screen: _____ inches
Can the monitor be raised / lowered? Y   N
Do you notice the screen flicker? Y   N
Does the screen have a glare filter? Y   N   If so, is it glass/mesh?
Top of display screen (above, equal to, below) eye level?
If above or below, by how many inches? _____

Workstation:

Viewing distance from your eye to keyboard: _____ inches
Viewing distance from your eye to hard copy material: _____ inches
Is the monitor supported on a (stand / desk / CPU)?

Visual Symptoms:

Do you experience any of the following symptoms during or after
computer work:

☐ Eyestrain   ☐ Double Vision
☐ Headaches   ☐ Neck ☐ Shoulder ☐ Wrist Ache
☐ Blurred Near Vision   ☐ Color Distortion
☐ Blurred Distant Vision ☐ Light Sensitivity
☐ Dry ☐ Irritated Eyes   ☐ Backache

Do you wear glasses while working at the computer?   Y   N
If yes, are they (single vision, bifocal, or progressive)?

Do you wear contact lenses while working at the computer? Y   N
If yes, are they (soft, gas permeable, or hard lenses)?

Appendix B

Seal of Acceptance Program for Computer Glare Reduction Filters

As of November 2004

The American Optometric Association (AOA) has established a program to provide evaluation and recognition of quality computer glare reduction filters. Products that meet the minimum specifications established by the AOA Commission on Ophthalmic Standards are allowed to use the AOA Seal of Acceptance in product labeling and marketing. Specifications for VDT/computer glare reduction filters cover construction quality, image quality, glare reduction, reflectance, and the ability to withstand environmental testing.

The following is a listing of companies whose products have met the AOA specifications for display screen glare reduction. You can contact these manufacturers directly for additional information about their filters.

Fellowes Manufacturing Company 630/893-1600
1789 Norwood Ave.
Itasca, IL 60143
www.fellowes.com

Accepted filter models: Premium Glass Anti-glare/Lite Tint, Premium Glass Anti-static/ Radiation/Lite Tint, Premium Glass Anti-glare/Traditional Tint, Premium Glass Anti-glare/Traditional Tint (Double sided coating), Premium Glass Anti-static/Radiation/Traditional Tint, Premium Contour Anti-glare/Lite Tint, Premium Contour Anti-static/Radiation/Lite Tint, Notebook Computer Anti-glare, and Glare 2000 Anti-Glare and Anti-Glare/Anti-Static/Radiation.

Kantek, Inc. 516/594-4600
3067 New St.
Oceanside, NY 11572
sales@kantek.com
www.kantek.com

Accepted filter models: Spectrum Universal and Spectrum Universal Contour.

Kensington Technology Group Division 800/535-4242
ACCO Brands, Inc.
2855 Campus Drive
San Mateo, CA 94403
www.kensington.com

Accepted filter models: Kensington High Contrast, Kensington True Color, GlareMaster Premium Contour and Flat Frame, GlareMaster Premium Anti-Radiation Contour and Flat Frame.

3M Safety and Security Systems Division 800/553-9215
3M Center, Bldg. 225-4N-14
St. Paul, MN 55144
www.3m.com

Accepted filter models: AF100/AF200, AF150/250, HF300, HF350, EF150, EF250, and PF400/500.

The AOA will regularly publish updated listings of accepted products. For additional information about the Seal of Certification and Acceptance program, contact the AOA Commission on Ophthalmic Standards, 243 N. Lindbergh Blvd., St. Louis, MO 63141, 314/991-4100, ext. 245.

Appendix C

Resources for the Blind and Visually Impaired

This list contains useful sources of information for blind and visually impaired computer users. The list is divided into four sections: Organizations; Newsletters and Journals; Networks, Bulletin Boards and Databases; and Books and Pamphlets. Please note that the list is based on information used in research and outreach programs. It is therefore likely that the list is not exhaustive. No recommendations or endorsements are implied by inclusion on this list.

Organizations

AFB Technology Center
American Foundation for the Blind, Inc.
11 Penn Plaza
Suite 300
New York, NY 10001
(212) 502-7642
(212) 502-7773 (FAX)
E-mail: techetr@aft.org

Conducts product evaluations of assistive technology including Braille technology, optical character readers, speech Trimesters, screen magnifiers, and closed circuit television.

American Council of the Blind
1155 15th Street, Suite 720
Washington, DC 20005
(202) 467-5081
(202) 467-5085 (FAX)

Publishes computer resource list about various devices and where to buy them. Visually Impaired Data Processors International, a computer users' special interest group, is part of ACB.

American Printing House for the Blind
PO Box 6085
1839 Frankfort Avenue
Louisville, KY 40206
(502) 895-2405
(800) 223-1939

Producers of software for users with visual impairments. APH also produces user manuals in Braille for Apple computers, instructional aids, tools, and supplies. Four-track recorder/players available. Tutorial kit for Microsoft Windows available for VI users.

Braille Institute
741 N. Vermont Avenue
Los Angeles, CA 90029
(323) 663-1111

This is an educational organization for persons who are blind, deaf-blind, or partially sighted. It has technological resources, a talking book library, and a large community outreach program. A subsidy program for funding equipment is available to persons who are currently employed and legally blind.

Carroll Center for the Blind
70 Centre Street
Newton, MA 02158
(617) 969-6200

Various publications and rehabilitation and educational programs are available for persons who are blind or visually impaired. A computer training program, Project CABLE, provides computer assessment, training on adaptive devices and software, and word processing training. Summer training courses for youth are also offered.

Central Blind Rehabilitation Center
Veterans Affairs
Edward Hines, Jr. VA Hospital
PO Box 5000 (124)
Hines, IL 60141-5000
(708) 216-2271

Information on various types of computer access devices for people with visual impairments.

Centre for Sight Enhancement
School of Optometry
University of Waterloo
Waterloo, ON N2L 3GI
CANADA
(519) 889-4708
(519) 746-2337 (FAX)

A clinical teaching and research facility providing assessment, prescription, instruction and/or rehabilitation by a multidisciplinary professional team. Provides sight enhancement devices under the Provincial Ministry of Health's Assistive Devices Program.

Helen Keller National Center for Deaf-Blind Youths and Adults
111 Middle Neck Road
Sands Point, NY 11050
(516) 944-8900
(516) 944-8637 (TTY)

Only national program that provides diagnostic evaluation. short-term comprehensive rehabilitation and personal adjustment training, and job preparation and placement for Americans who are deaf-blind. Local services provided through regional offices, affiliated agencies, a National Training Team, and a Technical Assistance Center for older adults.

International Braille and Technology Center for the Blind
National Center for the Blind
1800 Johnson Street
Baltimore, MD 21230
(410) 659-9314

Provides demonstrations, comparative evaluations, cost comparison, ADA compliance assistance, personal and telephone consultation pertaining to assistive technology for the visually impaired; tours meeting and conference facilities. Resource for blind persons and sighted individuals. Overnight and dining accommodations may be available for a fee.

National Association for Visually Handicapped
22 West 21ˢᵗ Street
New York, NY 10010
(212) 889-3141

Organization dealing with the needs of people who are partially sighted. Contact for information about computer access. Also a San Francisco office at 3201 Balboa Street, San Francisco, CA 94121.

National Braille Press, Inc.
88 St. Stephen Street
Boston, MA 02115
(617) 266-6160

Publications on personal computer technology for people who are blind. Many printer and modem manuals transcribed in Braille.

National Federation of the Blind
1800 Johnson Street
Baltimore, MD 21230
(410) 659-9314

Programs include: Committee on Evaluation of Technology (which evaluates current and proposed technology for people who are blind or visually impaired); International Braille and Technology Center for the Blind (a demonstration and evaluation center for computer technology for blind and visually impaired users); and NFB in Computer Science (a nationwide computer users' group which publishes an annual newsletter for people who are blind or visually impaired).

Newspapers for the Blind
DataCast Communications, Inc.
900 Lady Ellen Place Suite 23
Ottawa, ON KIZ 5L5
CANADA
(613) 725-2106
(613) 722-8756 (FAX)

Service that delivers an electronic version of Canada's well-known newspapers to computers via a VBI decoder attached to cable TV. Available newspapers are: Montreal Gazette, La Presse, Ottawa Citizen, Toronto Star, Toronto Sun, Financial Post, The Globe and Mail.

Recording for the Blind and Dyslexic (RFBD)
20 Rozel Road
Princeton, NJ 08540
(609) 221-4792
(609) 452-0606

Provides academic textbooks and other educational textbooks to people who cannot read standard print because of physical, perceptual, or other disabilities. Must be a registered member in order to borrow materials; call for details. Also sells reference books on disk and related software products.

Sensory Access Foundation
385 Sherman Avenue, Suite 2
Palo Alto, CA 94306
(650) 329-0430 (voice)
(650) 329-0433 (TDD)

Compiles and publishes consumer information on technology updates, including computer adaptations, for blind and visually impaired people. Assists in career placement for people who have visual impairments. Career services are only available within California; information services available worldwide. Publishes a magazine and has a technology training center.

Smith-Kettlewell Eye Research Institute
Rehabilitation Engineering Center
2232 Webster Street
San Francisco, CA 94115
(415) 561-1619

Research and development center on assistive technology (including work on computer access devices) for people who are blind or visually impaired.

Technology Center (TC)
American Foundation for the Blind
11 Penn Plaza
Suite 300
New York, NY 10001
(212) 502-7642
(800) 232-5463
E-mail: techtr@afb.org.

Conducts evaluations of assistive technology for visually impaired people and provides information on those products. Coordinates the Careers and Technology Information Bank (CTIB), a collection of data from visually impaired people who use adaptive equipment in a variety of jobs.

Newsletters and Journals

Braille Forum
American Council of the Blind
1155 15th Street
Suite 720
Washington, DC 20005
(202) 467-5081
(202) 467-5085 (FAX)

Publication dealing with blindness-related issues, such as legislation, technology, and product and service announcements.

Computer Folks
c/o Richard Ring
269 Terhune Avenue
Passaic, NJ 07055
(201) 471-4211

A magazine on cassette for blind computer users by blind computer users. Discusses and demonstrates adaptive technology.

Journal of Visual Impairment and Blindness
American Federation for the Blind
11 Penn Plaza
Suite 300
New York, NY 10001
(212) 502-7600

Research journal on issues related to visual impairment and blindness. Includes research reviews, application papers, and articles on special topics (including assistive technology). Published monthly, except July and August.

Tactic
Clovernook Center
7000 Hamilton Avenue
Cincinnati, OH 45231
(513) 522-3860

International quarterly offers information and reviews on technology for people with visual impairments. Published in Braille, large print, and diskette (IBM compatible) formats.

Technology Update
Sensory Access Foundation
385 Sherman Avenue, Suite #2
Palo Alto, CA 94306
(650) 329-0430 (voice)
(650) 329-0433 (TDD)

Bimonthly newsletter with information regarding technology and vision impairment. Includes new product announcements, product reviews, and consumer information. Available in print, large print, cassette, and PC diskette.

Visual Field
Florida Instructional Materials Center
5002 North Lois Avenue
Tampa, FL 33614
(813) 872-5281
(813) 872-5284 (FAX)

Biannual newsletter on products, projects, conferences, etc., related to education of students with visual impairments.

Networks, Bulletin Boards, and Databases

4 Sights Network
Upshaw Institute for the Blind
16625 Grand River
Detroit, MI 48227
(313) 272-3900
(313) 272-7111 (dial in)

This computer network provides bulletin board and database information for blind and visually impaired individuals and those working with them. The information covers vocational and rehabilitation resources, assistive technology, educational information for parents, teachers, and students, public policy and more.

Carl et Al
American Printing House for the Blind
Attn: Paul Brown
PO Box 6085
Louisville, KY 40206-0085
(800) 223-1939
(502) 895-1509 (FAX)

An on-line database that lists materials in media accessible to people who are visually impaired. Over 120,000 records including Braille books, large type materials, music scores, electronic books, sound recordings, software programs, and tactile graphics. Contact APH for billing and access information.

Books and Pamphlets

CD-ROM Advantage
D. Croft, D. Kendrick, and A. Gayzagian (1994)
National Braille Press
88 St. Stephen Street
Boston, MA 02115
(617) 266-6160
(617) 437-0456 (FAX)

Answers commonly asked questions about CD-ROM technology and how it works with speech and Braille. Includes practical advice from users, profiles blind users of CD-ROM, and lists over 100 CD-ROM titles.

Computer Access, Resource Manual
Rosenbaum, et al. (1987)
Carroll Center for the Blind
770 Centre Street
Newton, MA 02158
   (617) 969-6200

Resource manual and curriculum for setting up an evaluation and training center in assistive technology applications for blind and visually impaired.

Customer Service Representative Training Manual
Ferrarin, Rosenbaum, et al. (1994)
Carroll Center for the Blind
770 Centre Street
Newton, MA 02158
(617) 969-6200

A comprehensive curriculum for creating and providing job readiness skills for employment in customer service jobs to individuals with visual impairments utilizing assistive technology. For rehabilitation agencies, secondary institutions, or career counselors.

Extend Their Reach
Electronic Industries Association
2500 Wilson Boulevard
Arlington, VA 22201
(703) 907-7600

Gives introduction to the types of products available to overcome impairments of sight, speech, hearing, motion, etc. Also provides information on how to find funding for and producers of assistive devices, listing of companies, and resources for further information.

Job Readiness Workshop
Carroll Center for the Blind
770 Centre Street
Newton, MA 02158
(617) 969-6200

Step by step guide on creating a resume and developing interviewing techniques. Sample resumes and example interview questions given.

Medical Transcription Training Manual
Ferrarini, Rosenbaum, et al. (1994)
Carroll Center for the Blind
770 Centre Street
Newton, NM 02158
(617) 969-6200

Curriculum, guidelines, and resources for creating or modifying medical transcription programs for persons with visual disabilities. The 180 page manual includes detailed course outlines for terminology, transcription and computer instruction, resources, job information.

Print and Braille Literacy: Selecting Appropriate Learning Media
Hilda Caton, Ed.D.
American Printing House for the Blind, Inc.
1839 Frankfort Avenue
PO Box 6085
Louisville, KY 40206
(502) 895-2405

Provides guidelines designed to ensure that every visually impaired student will have adequate opportunity for learning to use the medium/media most appropriate for his or her needs. Guidelines were developed by a committee of experts in the field.

Project CABLE Resource Manual, 2nd edition (1987)
Project CABLE (Computer Access for the Blind in Education and Employment)
Carroll Center for the Blind
770 Centre Street
Newton, MA 02158
(617) 969-6200

This manual includes curriculum, evaluation form, lesson plans, and other resources to assist in setting up or running an employment program for persons who are blind or visually impaired. Other topics include funding and staffing.

TeleSelling Training Manual
Carroll Center for the Blind
770 Centre Street
Newton, MA 02158
(617) 969-6200

Curriculum, guidelines, and resources for creating or modifying a telemarketing training program for persons with visual disabilities. Chapters included information about the field, developing a program, tele-selling skills, computer course outlines, job readiness workshop.

Tools for Selecting Appropriate Learning Media
American Printing House for the Blind
PO Box 6095
1839 Frankfort Avenue
Louisville, KY 40206-0085
(800) 223-1839

An extension of the book Print and Braille Literacy. *Designed to help parents, teachers, and administrators make decisions concerning students' use of Braille, print, or both as their primary reading medium/media.*

Vendor Information Sheets
Consumer Information Department of Sensory Access Foundation
385 Sherman Avenue, Suite 2
Palo Alto, CA 94306
(650) 329-0430
(650) 323-1062 (FAX)

List vendor names, addresses, phone numbers, fax numbers, BBSs and prices for access products for people who are blind or low vision. Sheets available for: screen readers, speech synthesizers, computer magnification closed circuit televisions, Braille devices and software, reading machines, and others.

Appendix D

*Computer Access Products for Blind
and Visually Impaired Users*

Listed below are makers of products which allow blind and visually impaired people to use computers. The three types of output which these systems use are: synthesized speech, large print, and Braille or other tactile output. The products listed may consist of hardware, software, or a combination. Braille printers are also included in this list. Most of these products are designed to provide access to standard commercial software (word processors, spreadsheets, etc.) designed for the nondisabled marketplace. A few are dedicated programs, specifically designed for people with visual impairments, but not providing access to other software.

These addresses are provided so you can find out what's available. We suggest you contact the companies for more information, and that you also do some investigating on your own, such as reading books or magazines, talking to users of the products, searching the internet, or consulting experts on the topic.

Access Systems International, LTD
415 English Avenue
Monterey, CA 93940
(831) 375-5313
Braille Access
Index Basic
Index Basic-D
Index Everest-D

ADA Compliance Information
US Department of Justice
(800) 514-0301
(800) 514-0383 (TDD)
http://www.usdoj.gov/crt/ada/
adahom1.htm

AI Squared
P.O. Box 669
Manchester Center, VT 05255-0669
(802) 362-3612
FAX (802) 362-1670
ZoomText

American Printing House for the Blind
 (APH)
P.O. Box 6085
Louisville, KY 40206-0085
(502) 895-2405
(800) 223-1839
Braille 'n Speak Classic
Echo II with Textalker & Echo II with
Textalker-GSNOMAD Talking Touch
 Pad & NOMAD Gold
Speaqualizer Speech Access System
TEXTALKER
Textalker-GS

American Thermoform Corporation
2311 Travers Avenue
City of Commerce, CA 90040
(323) 723-9021
Braille 200
Braille 400 S
Braille Comet
KTS Braille Display
Ohtsuki BT-5000 Braille/Print Printer

Apple Computer, Inc.
Worldwide Disability Solutions
 Group, MS
38DS. I Infinite Loop
Cupertino, CA 95014
(408) 600-7808
TT/TDD (800) 755-0601
applesdsg@eworld.com
www.apple.com/disability/
CloseView

Arkenstone, Inc.
1390 Borregas Avenue
Sunnyvale, CA 94089
(800) 444 4443
(408) 752-2200
TT/TDD (800) 833-2753
info@arkenstone.org
Open Book
Open Book Unbound

Artic Technologies
55 Park Street
Troy, MI 48083
(248) 588-7370
FAX (810) 588-2650
Artic TransBook
Artic TransType
Business Vision
Gizmo
Magnum Deluxe
Magnum GT
Win Vision

ATR/JWA, Inc.
P.O. Box 180
Fairfax Station, VA 22039
(703) 715-6072
FAX (703) 903-9142
BRAILLEX-2D
Notex 486

Berkeley Systems, Inc.
2095 Rose St.
Berkeley, CA 94709
(510) 540-5535 ext. 716
TT/TDD (510) 849-9426
osw@berksys.com
inLARGE 2.0
outSPOKEN 1.7
outSPOKEN for Windows

Biolink Computer Research
 and Development, LTD
Suite 105 - 140 West 15th
North Vancouver, BC
V7M IR6 CANADA
(604) 984-4099
BBS (604) 985-8431
FAX (604) 985-8493
Protalk23 for Windows

B-K Press of Texas
P.O. Box 4843
Wichita Falls, TX 76308
(817) 723-0254 FAX
http://www.theshoppes.com/
~bkpress

Blazie Engineering
105 East Jarrettsville Road
Forest Hill, MD 21050
(410) 893-9333
BBS (410) 893-8944
FAX (410) 836-5040
info@blazie.com
http://blazie.com/
Braille 'n Speak
Braille Blazer
Braille Lite
Type 'n Speak

Carolyn's
Box 14577
Bradenton, FL. 34820-4577
(800) 648-2266
FAX (813) 761-8306

Compusult Limited
40 Bannister Street
P.O. Box 1000
Mount Pearl, NF AlN 3C9 CANADA
(709) 745-7914
FAX (709) 745-7927
scantell@compusult.nf.ca
www.compusult.nf.ca
ScanTELL

Duxbury Systems, Inc.
435 King Street
Littleton, MA 01460
(508) 486-9766

Easier Ways, Inc.
1101 N. Calvert Street, Suite 405
Baltimore, MD. 21202
(410) 659-0232 / (410) 659-0233 (FAX)

Enabling Technologies Company
3102 S.E. Jay Street
Stuart, FL 34997
(800) 777-3687
FAX (407) 220-2920
Braille BookMaker and Braille Express
 100 & 500
Juliet Brailler
Marathon Brailler
Romeo Brailer Model RB-25
Romeo Brailler Model RB-40
Thomas Brailler
TranSend System

Equipment for Visually Disabled
 People: An International Guide
Technical Research and Development
 Department
Royal National Institute for the Blind
224 Great Portland Street
London WI N 6 AA, England

Florida New Concepts Marketing, Inc.
P.O. Box 261, Port Richey, FL 34673
(813) 842-3231
FAX (813) 845-7544
Beamscope
Compu-Lenz

Franklin Electronic Publishers, Inc.
Franklin Learning Resources Division
One Franklin Plaza
Burlington, NJ 08016-4907
(800) 525-9673
(609) 386-2500
Language Master Special Edition
LM6000SE

General Services Administration
Center for Information Technology
  Accommodation
18th & F Street, NW
Room 1234
Washington, DC 20405
202-501-4906 (Voice)
(202) 501-2010 (TTY)
(202) 501-6269 (FAX)

GW Micro
310 Racquet Drive
Fort Wayne, IN 46825
(219) 483-3625
FAX (219) 482-2492
support@gwmicro.com
Vocal-Eyes
Window-Eyes

Henter-Joyce, Inc.
2100 62nd Avenue North
St. Petersburg, FL 33702
(800) 336-5658
(813) 528-8900
BBS (813) 528-8903
FAX (813) 528-8901
7477.3306@compuserve.com
JAWS for Windows
JAWS Screenreader
WordScholar

Hexagon Products
P.O. Box 1295
Park Ridge, IL 60068
(708) 692-3355
76064.1776@compuserve.com
B-Pop
Big-W

HumanWare, Inc.
6245 King Road
Loomis, CA 95650
(800) 722-3393
(708) 620-0722
FAX (916) 652-7296
ALVA Braille Terminals
Braille-N-Print
Keynote Companion
MasterTOUCH
Mountbatten Brailler
Paragon Braille Printer
Ransley Braille Interface (RBI)
Soundproof

IBM Corporation
Special Needs Systems
P.O. Box 1328
Internal Zip 5432
Boca Raton, FL 33432
(800) 426-4832
TT/TDD (800) 426-4833
EBM Screen Reader/2
IBM Screen Reader/DOS
Screen Magnifier/2

Innoventions, Inc.
5921 S. Middlefield Road, Suite 102
Littleton, CO 80123
(800) 854-6554
http://www.magnicam.com/magni-
cam/

Kansys, Inc.
4301 Wimbledon Ter. 2B
Lawrence, KS 66047
(913) 843-0351
PROVOX

Konz, Ned
810 21st Avenue North
St. Petersburg, FL 33704
nedkonz@gate.net,
76046.223@compuserve.com
Lens 2.03

Less Gauss Inc.
Suite 160
187 East Market Street
Rhinebeck, NY 12572
(800) 872-1051
(914) 876-5432
FAX (914) 876-2005
Adjustable EZ Magnifier
GNK Magnifier
NuVu Magnifier

Lighthouse Enterprises
Consumer Products Division
36-20 Northern Blvd.
Long Island City, NY 11101
(800) 829-0500

LS & S Group
P.O. Box 673
Northbrook, IL 60065
(800) 468-4789 or (800) 708-498-9777

Massachusetts Association for the
 Blind
200 Ivy Street
Brookline, MA 02146-3995
(617) 738-5110/ In Mass. (800) 682-9200
TDD (617) 731-6444/FAX (617) 738-1247

Mayer-Johnson Company
P.O. Box 1579
Solana Beach, CA 92075
(858) 550-0084
FAX (858) 550-0084
mayerj@aol.com
Infovox 210

Microsystems Software Inc.
600 Worcester Road
Framingham, MA 01701
(800) 828-2600
(508) 879-9000
BBS (508) 875-8009
FAX (508) 626-8515
HandiCHAT and HandiCHAT Deluxe
MAGic and MAGic Deluxe

MicroTalk Software
917 Clear Creek Drive
Texarkana, TX 75503
(903) 832-3471
Modem (903) 832-3722
FAX (903) 832-3722
ASAP (Automatic Speech Access
 Program)

MONS International, Inc.
Products for the Visually Impaired
6595 Roswell Road #224
Atlanta, GA 30328
(800) 541-7903
(404) 551-8455

National Institute for Rehabilitation
 Engineering
P.O. Box T
Hewitt, NJ 07421
(800) 736-2216
(201) 853-6585
dons@warwick.net
Large-Type Display Utility Software

New Concepts Marketing
P.O. Box 261
Port Richey, FL 34673
(800) 456-7097

Okay Vision-Aide Corporation
14811 Myford Rd.
Tustin, CA 92680
(800) 325-4488
E-mail: vision-aide@ovac.com

OMS Development
610-B Forest Avenue
Wilmette, IL 60091
(708) 251-5787
(800) 831-0272
FAX (708) 251-5793
ebholman@metcom.com
Tinytalk

Optelec USA, Inc.
6 Lyberty Way
P.O. Box 729
Westford, MA 01886
(800) 828-1056
(508) 392-0767
LP-DOS & LP-Windows

The Productivity Works, Inc.
7 Belmont Circle
Trenton, NJ 08618
(609) 984-8044
(609) 984-8048
www.prodworks.com

S. Walter, Inc.
30423 Canwood St., Suite 115
Agoura Hills, CA 91301
(818) 406-2202
(800) 992-5837

Science Products for the Blind
P.O. Box 888
Southeastern, PA 19399
(800) 888-7400

Sigma Designs, Inc.
47906 Bayside Parkway
Fremont, CA 94538
(510) 770-0100

Speech Systems for the Blind
76 Wheaton Drive
Attleboro, MA 02703
(508) 226-0447
73030.3644@compuserve.com
Seekline
WINKLINE

Syntha-Voice Computers Inc.
9009-1925 Pine Street
Niagra Falls, NY 14301
(905) 662-0565
(800) 263-4540
BBS (905) 662-0569
FAX (905) 662-0568
help@synthavoice.on.ca
Panorama
Powerama
Slimware
Slimware Window Bridge

Technology for Independence
529 Main Street
Schraft Center Annex
Boston, MA 02129
(617) 242-7007

Telephone Pioneers of America
P.O. Box 18388
Denver, CO 80204
(303) 571-1200

TeleSensory Corporation
455 North Bernardo Avenue
P.O. Box 7455
Mountain View, CA 94039
(650) 960-0920
(800) 804-8004
BrailleMate 2
David
DM80/FM
INKA
Optacon II
PowerBraille 40, 65. & 80
ScreenPower
ScreenPower for Windows
Vantage CCD
VersaPoint-40 Braille Embosser
Vista

TFi Engineering
529 Main Street
Boston, MA 02129
(800) 843-6962
(617) 242-7007
FAX (617) 242-2007
Myna

Trace R&D Center
S-151 Waisman Center
1500 Highland Avenue
Madison, WI 53705
(608) 263-2309
TDD: (608) 263-5408

T.V. Raman
(617) 692-7637
raman@crl.dec.com
http://www.cr.dec.com/crl/people/
 biographies/
raman.html
Emacspeak

VisuAide
841 Jean-Paul Vincent
 Boulevard
Longueuil, PQ J4G IR3
CANADA
(514) 463-1717
FAX (514) 463-0120
Magnum

Xerox Imaging Systems, Inc.
9 Centennial Drive
Peabody, MA 01960
(800) 248-6550
BookWise
Reading AdvantEdge

Appendix E

Additional Resources

American College of Occupational and
  Environmental Medicine (**ACOEM)**
1114 N. Arlington Heights Road
Arlington Heights, IL, 60004-4770
Telephone: (847) 818-1800
FAX: (847) 818-9266
www.acoem.org

American Industrial Hygiene
  Association (AIHA)
2700 Prosperity Avenue, Suite 250
Fairfax, VA 22031
(703) 849-8888
FAX: (703) 207-3561
www.aiha.org
E-mail: infonet@aiha.org

American National Standards Institute
  (ANSI)
1819 L Street, NW, 6th floor
Washington, DC 20036
Tel: (202) 293-8020
FAX: (202) 293-9287
www.ansi.org

American Optometric Association
243 North Lindbergh Blvd.
St. Louis, MO 63141
(314) 991-4100
FAX: (314) 991-4101
www.aoa.org

American Society of Safety Engineers
1800 East Oakton Street
Des Plaines, IL 60018-2187
(847) 699-2929
www.asse.org

American Society of Testing and
  Materials (ASTM)
100 Barr Harbor Drive
P.O. Box C700
West Conshohocken, PA 19428-2959
(610) 832-9585
FAX: (610) 832-9555
www.astm.org

College of Optometrists in Vision
  Development
243 N. Lindbergh Blvd., Ste #310
St. Louis, MO 63141 USA
(314) 991-4007 or (888) 268-3770
(314) 991-1167 (FAX)
E-mail: info@covd.org

Corporate Vision Consulting
The Eye-CEE System for Computer
  Users®
842 Arden Drive
Encinitas, CA 92024
(800) 383-1202 (Voice/FAX)
E-mail: eyedoc@adnc.com
www.cvconsulting.com

Dept. of Health and Human Resources
200 Independence Ave., SW
Washington, DC 20201
202-619-0257
877-696-6775
www.os.dhhs.gov

Department of Labor
200 Constitution Ave., NW
Washington, DC 20210
202-219-7316
www.dol.gov

Equal Employment Opportunity
  Commission (ADA)
1801 L Street, NW
Washington, DC 20507
202-663-4900
www.eeoc.gov

Human Factors and Ergonomic Society
P O Box 1369
Santa Monica, CA 90406-1369
310-394-1811
www.hfes.org
E-mail: info@hfes.org

Illuminating Engineering Society
  (IESNA)
120 Wall Street, Floor 17
New York, NY 10005
212-248-5000
FAX: 212-248-5017/18
www.iesna.org
E-mail: iesna@iesna.org

National Institute for Occupational
  Safety and Health (NIOSH)
Centers for Disease Control
1600 Clifton Road, NE
Atlanta, GA 30333
404-639-3534
www.cdc.gov/niosh/homepage.html

National Safety Council
1121 Spring Lake Drive
Itasca, IL 60143-3201
708-285-1121
www.nsc.org

Occupational Safety and Health
  Administration (OSHA)
US Dept. of Labor
200 Constitution Avenue, NW
Washington, DC 20216
800-282-1048
www.osha.gov

Optometric Extension Program
  Foundation, Inc.
2912 South Daimler
Santa Ana, CA 92705
949-250-8070
www.oep.org

Prevent Blindness America
500 E. Remington Road
Schaumburg, IL 60173
800-331-2020
www.preventblindness.org

Vision Council of America
1700 Diagonal Rd, Ste. 500
Alexandria, VA 22314
703-548-4560
www.checkyearly.com

Glossary

Accommodation   In regard to the visual system, the focusing ability of the eye.

Acuity   A measure of the ability of the eye to resolve fine detail, specifically to distinguish that two points separated in space are distinctly separate.

Astigmatism   A visual condition in which the light entering the eye is distorted such that it does not focus at one single point in space.

Behavioral optometry   A branch of optometry based on a model of vision that addresses a holistic approach to visual function, stating that vision and visual abilities can be trained or enhanced.

Binocularity   The use of two eyes at the same time, where the usable visual areas of each eye overlap to produce a three-dimensional perception.

Brightness   The subjective attribute of light to which humans assign a label between very dim and very bright (brilliant). Brightness is perceived, not measured. Brightness is what is perceived when lumens fall on the rods and cones of the eye's retina. The sensitivity of the eye decreases as the magnitude of the light increases, and the rods and cones are sensitive to the luminous energy per unit of time (power) impinging on them.

Cataracts   A loss of clarity of the crystalline lens within the eye that causes partial or total blindness.

Cathode ray tube (CRT)   A glass tube that forms part of earlier video display terminals. The tube generates a stream of electrons that strike the phosphor-coated display screen and cause light to be emitted. The light forms characters on the screen.

Color convergence   Alignment of the three electron beams in the CRT that generate the three primary screen colors — red, green and blue — used to form images on screen. In a misconverged image, edges will have color fringes (for example, a white area might have a blue fringe on one side).

Color temperature   A way of measuring color accuracy. Adjusting a monitor's color-temperature control, for example, may change a bluish white to a whiter white.

Convergence   The visual function of realigning the eyes to attend an object closer than optical infinity. The visual axes of the eyes continually point closer to each other, as the object of viewing gets closer to the viewer.

Computer vision syndrome (CVS)   The complex of eye and vision problems related to near work that are experienced during or related to computer use.

Diplopia (double vision)   That visual condition in which the person experiences two distinct images while looking at one object. This results from the breakdown of the person's coordination skills.

Dot matrix   A pattern of dots that forms characters (text) or constructs a display image (graphics) on the display screen.

Dot pitch   The distance between two phosphor dots of the same color on the screen.

Dynamic random access memory (DRAM)   (Pronounced DEE-ram) The readable/writable memory used to store data in personal computers. DRAM stores each bit of information in a cell composed of a capacitor and a transistor. Because the capacitor in a DRAM cell can hold a charge for only a few milliseconds, DRAM must be continually refreshed in order to retain its data.

Electromagnetic radiation   A form of energy resulting from electric and magnetic effects that travel as invisible waves.

Ergonomics   The study of the relationship between humans and their work. The goal of ergonomics is to increase worker comfort, productivity, and safety.

Eyesight   The process of receiving light rays into the eyes and focusing them onto the retina for interpretation.

Eyestrain (asthenopia)   Descriptive terms for symptoms of visual discomfort. Symptoms include burning, itching, tiredness, aching, watering, blurring, etc.

Farsightedness (hyperopia)   A visual condition where objects at a distance are more easily focused, as opposed to objects up close.

Focal length   The distance from the eye to the viewed object needed to obtain clear focus.

Font   A complete set of characters, including typeface, style, and size, used for screen or printer displays.

Hertz (HZ)   Cycles per second. Used to express the refresh rate of CRT displays.

Holistic   An attempt to see the whole situation and to treat the person, not as individual parts, but as a whole performance system.

Illuminance   The luminous flux incident on a surface per unit area. The unit is the lux, or lumen per square meter. The foot-candle (fc), or lumen per square foot is also used. An illuminance photometer measures the luminous flux per unit area at the surface being illuminated without regard to the direction from which the light approaches the sensor.

Interlaced An interlaced monitor scans the odd lines of an image first, followed by the even lines. This scanning method does not successfully eliminate flicker on computer screens.

Lag In optometric terms, the measured difference between the viewed object and the actual focusing distance.

Light The radiant energy that is capable of exciting the retina and producing a visual sensation. The visible wavelengths of the electromagnetic spectrum extend from about 380 to 770 nm. The unit of light energy is the lumen.

Liquid crystal display (LCD) A display technology that relies on polarizing filters and liquid-crystal cells rather than phosphors illuminated by electron beams to produce an on-screen image. To control the intensity of the red, green, and blue dots that comprise pixels, an LCD's control circuitry applies varying charges to the liquid-crystal cells through which polarized light passes on its way to the screen.

Luminance The luminous intensity per unit area projected in a given direction. The unit is the candela per square meter, which is still sometimes called a nit. The footlambert (fL) is also in common use. Luminance is the measurable quantity that most closely corresponds to brightness.

Luminous flux Visible power, or light energy, per unit of time. It is measured in lumens. Since light is visible energy, the lumen refers only to visible power.

Luminous intensity The luminous flux per solid angle emitted or reflected from a point. The unit of measure is the lumen per steradian, or candela (cd). (The steradian is the unit of measurement of a solid angle.)

Macular degeneration A degenerative condition in which loss of central vision occurs. Usually occurs later in life (also referred to as age-related macular degeneration, or AMD).

MegaHertz (MHz) A measurement of frequency in millions of cycles per second.

Mouse A computer input device connected to the CPU.

Musculoskeletal Relating to the muscles and skeleton of the human body.

Myopia (near-sightedness) The ability to see objects clearly only at a close distance.

Nearpoint   The common near point of viewing, usually within arms length.

Noninterlaced   A noninterlaced monitor scans the lines of an image sequentially, from top to bottom. This method provides less visible flicker than interlaced scanning.

Ocular motility   Relating to the movement abilities of the eyes.

On-screen controls   On-screen controls let you change settings as you would program a VCR. Visual feedback is provided on-screen as you push certain buttons.

Perception   The understanding of sensory input (vision, hearing, touch, etc.).

Phosphor   A substance that emits light when stimulated by electrons.

Pixel   The smallest element of a display screen that can be independently assigned color and intensity.

Polarity   The arrangement of the light and dark images on the screen. Normal polarity has light characters against a dark background; Reverse polarity has dark characters against a light background.

Presbyopia   A reduction in the ability to focus on near objects caused by the decreased flexibility in the lens, usually due to the person being over 40 years old.

Presets   Many monitors offer control presets that enable you to switch between different resolutions and color depths. The number of custom settings varies from monitor to monitor, and ranges from around 4 to 28 settings.

Random access memory (RAM)   The generic term for read/write memory — memory that permits bits and bytes to be written to it as well as read from it — used in modern computers.

Refractive   Having to do with the bending of light rays, usually in producing a sharp optical image.

Refresh rate   The number of times per second that the screen phosphors must be painted to maintain proper character display.

Resolution   The number of pixels, horizontally and vertically, that make up a screen image. The higher the resolution, the more detailed the image.

Resting point of accommodation (RPA)   The point in space where the eyes naturally focus when at rest.

Suppression   The "turning off" of the image of one eye by the brain, most often to avoid double vision or reduce excess stress.

Swim   A wave-like motion of screen display information, usually in a vertical direction, due to electrical malfunctioning in the monitor.

Video display terminal (VDT)   An electronic device consisting of a monitor unit (e.g., cathode ray tube) with which to view input into a computer.

Vision   A learned awareness and perception of visual experiences (combined with any or all other senses) that results in mental or physical action. Not simply eyesight.

Vision therapy   A treatment (by behavioral optometrists) used to develop and enhance visual abilities.

Visual stress   The inability of a person to visually process light information in a comfortable, efficient manner.

VRAM (video RAM)   (Pronounced VEE-ram) A dual-ported RAM design that lets the memory chip read and write simultaneously. The higher throughput results in higher resolution and color modes. VRAM enables a block write feature, which is useful for handling video.

Index